EAT, SLEEP, RELAX, PROTECT, FORGET

ALSO BY MICHELLE SEXTON

**CANNABIS USE SURVEY:
CONFESSIONS, INSIGHTS, AND OPINIONS**
(with Dr. Laurie K. Mischley, 2016, Coffeetown Press)

Eat, Sleep, Relax, Protect, Forget is a treasure chest of priceless information. In a refreshing fashion that is professional, practical, and personal, Dr. Sexton shares her intimate knowledge of the endocannabinoid system as well as holistic healing, guiding us all on a path to wellness. She presents complex well-researched science in an easily digestible fashion—honest and human. The illustrative cases, herbal allies and yoga chakra associations facilitate our ability to put the elegant science to work in our journey towards thriving.

—**Donald I. Abrams, MD,** *Integrative Oncologist, UCSF Osher Center for Integrative Health, Professor Emeritus of Medicine, University of California San Francisco*

"So many women, myself included, have chronic health issues we've been told have no real treatments. If you've been searching for solutions beyond just living with the pain, this book is for you.

Eat, Sleep, Relax, Forget, Protect is a phenomenally helpful guide for women looking to improve their well-being by improving endocannabinoid function. The book delves into the science of the endocannabinoid system and how it impacts women's health, while also giving helpful suggestions on how to help it heal and thrive. Beyond just advice on using cannabis for healing, this guide offers a variety of other natural methods like herbal remedies, yoga, and mindfulness, to restore our endocannabinoid system to a healthy place."

—**Emily Earlenbaugh, PhD** *is a journalist and educator and a regular contributor* Forbes

"In *Eat, Sleep, Relax, Protect, Forget,* Dr. Michelle Sexton takes a walk through the Endocannabinoid System from a unique perspective of THE WHOLE PATIENT! . . .the way we ALL should practice medicine! I love the way she carefully weaves the ECS and its functional elements with body/mind activity, women's health related functions and other general disorders. She then wraps the research-based descriptions in brilliant and personal discussions of the complimentary approaches: terpenes, herbal allies and a fantastic take on the chakras to complete the cycle. It's a reader-friendly venerable self-help book for cannabis use for wellness in 2023 that MEN and WOMEN should read!!!

—**Genester Wilson-King, MD FACOG,***Medical Director Victory Rejuvenation Center, Lake Mary FL,*

Eat, Sleep, Relax, Protect, Forget—are action words chosen by researcher Vincenzo Di Marzo in 1998 to describe the recently discovered endocannabinoid system (ECS). Dr. Michelle Sexton has brilliantly used those words as chapter headings to describe this incredibly complex molecular signaling system's role in helping us attain, maintain and/or regain health or homeostasis. This book not only helps us understand how the ECS functions throughout our bodies and why cannabis has such a wide range of therapeutic value, but it also provides guidance in the care and feeding of the ECS to promote individual health. This is a great book for those who strive for optimal health and a must read for nurses whose primary purpose is to help patients heal and achieve optimal wellness.

> —**Mary Lynn Mathre, RN,** *MSN Founding Member, American Cannabis Nurses Association and the Academy of Cannabis Education*

EAT
SLEEP
RELAX
PROTECT
FORGET

An Endocannabinoid (ECS)
Guide to Systems Wholeness
for Women

MICHELLE SEXTON, ND

Eat, Sleep, Relax, Protect, Forget: An Endocannabinoid (ECS) Guide to Systems Wholeness for Women

© 2023, Michelle Sexton. All rights reserved.

Published by Wayfaring Woman Publishing, San Diego, California

ISBN 979-8-9887864-0-5 (paperback)

ISBN 979-8-9887864-1-2 (eBook)

Library of Congress Control Number: 2023917261

Website: ecsdoctor.com | Instagram: @dr.michellesexton

This book contains advice and information related to health care. It should be used to supplement and not replace the advice of your doctor or another trained health professional. It is recommended that you seek your physician's advice before embarking on any medical program or treatment, particularly if you know or suspect that you have a health problem. All efforts have been made to ensure the accuracy of the information contained in this book as of the date of publication. This publisher and author disclaim liability for any medical outcomes that may occur as a result of applying the methods suggested in this book.

Publication managed by AuthorImprints.com

Contents

Figures and Illustrations

Introduction

This book is intended to help you adapt: to thrive rather than merely survive. It intends to clear up confusion, unravel **herban legends**, and provide evidence-based information to help you use an integrative toolkit to enhance your health. You will understand what a whole person approach is and how to wield it to enhance your health. The endocannabinoid system (referred to going forward as simply the ECS) will be your guide.

Eat, sleep, relax, protect, forget (recombined here) is a phrase coined by an ECS researcher Vincenzo Di Marzo, published in a paper in 1998.[1] The paper hypothesized: "Thus, 'relax, eat, sleep, forget and protect' might be some of the messages that are produced by the actions of endocannabinoids (ECBs: our naturally occuring cannabinoid compounds—yes named after the cannabis plant), alone or in combination with other mediators." Di Marzo speculated that ECBs have a general function as stress-recovery factors. These roles of the ECS to provide that we eat, sleep, relax, protect, and forget are all survival-based. The ECS modulates signaling across all of our tissues and signaling pathways. This book outlines the ECS and provides information on how it can be used as a systems biology approach for stress recovery, for addressing homeostasis of systems, and for health, healing and well-being.

If you feel confused about cannabis, you are not alone! Because of the marginalization of the cannabis plant, healthcare providers have had inadequate experience or training around the benefits and harms of use. This is not uncommon for a botanical medicine since the study of phytochemicals (plant chemicals) is the domain of naturopathic medicine and herbalism. Enthusiasts of cannabis are perpetuating marketing claims yet may not fully understand there is a lack of evidence to back up perceived health benefits.

Researchers spent many years searching to uncover the primary active ingredient in cannabis. Finally, in 1964 Professor Raphael Mechoulam's laboratory isolated delta-9-tetrahydrocannabinol (THC) from cannabis.[2] This discovery unleashed sixty years of research into the actions and effects of this unique phytochemical and others like it. Why do we have a protein receptor for a plant chemical? It is because of our natural evolution alongside plants. Our bodies make the endogenous messengers that originate from within (the ECBs) that THC mimics. There are many plants that produce cannabinoid compounds and they will be referred to as plant cannabinoids (PCBs).

The ECS is composed of the endocannabinoid compounds that are lipid (fat-loving) transmitters; the protein receptors that interact with them; and the enzymes that make them and break them down. Collectively, the protein receptors (or cannabinoid receptors, CBR) identified for their coupling to (or binding) THC are called CB1 and CB2. The endogenous compounds that activate them were named anandamide, from Ananda the Sanskrit word for bliss (aka AEA), and 2-arachidonoylglycerol (aka 2AG).[3] The blissful AEA chemical is what our bodies use in the short term to help us respond to stressful situations. It is often involved in feedback loops, as the ECS is able to communicate across tissues.

In the amygdala, a deep brain structure, our stress-related nerves are monitored and AEA helps them regulate. 2AG[4] also binds to and activates both CB1R and CB2R, and is considered to be the more prominent endocannabinoid at work in the brain.

BOX 1.1   PROTEIN RECEPTORS: Chemical receptors are proteins, built from amino acids, and function by receiving and transducing our biological signals using chemical messengers. Protein receptors are found both inside and outside surfaces of cells and circulating in the blood. CBRs are seven transmembrane receptors, meaning the protein chains pass through the cell membrane 7 times. Internal to the cell, they are coupled to a messaging system known as G proteins, there-fore called G protein-coupled receptors (GPCRs). About 15 years after THC was isolated CB1 was discovered in 2 labs in the 1980s. CBRs bind cannabinoids, whether they are made from a plant, synthesized in a lab or made within our bodies as endocannabinoids.

The enzymes that synthesize and break down* ECBs are important in reg-ulating the physiology of all mammals. The ECBs are both in families of related compounds that also uses these enzymes.

CB1R is the most highly expressed receptor of its type in the brain, CB1R is also found outside of the brain, in nerves, skeletal muscle, fat, liver, heart, and smooth muscles (that encircles our blood vessels and intestines). The CB2R is primarily found in immune cells and plays a generous role in lim-iting chronic inflammation. It may be expressed on some nerve cells and is also found inside the cell. CB2R can be carried into the brain on the cell surface of immune cells migrating into the brain during inflammation. It can also be upregulated in the immune cells are already living in the brain (microglia) during inflammation.

Why have I only mentioned the plant cannabinoid THC and not canna-bidiol (CBD), the other major plant cannabinoid that seems to have taken the world by storm? THC directly activates both CBRs. There is misinfor-mation about CBD due to a relative lack of research in humans compared to that of THC. Many CBD marketing claims have not been backed up by formal study. While CBD may bind to CBRs, it does not activate them and

---

* The biosynthetic enzymes for ECBs are biosynthetic enzymes: N-acyl phosphati-dylethanolamine phospholipase D (NAPE-PLD), diacylglycerol lipase-α (DAGLα), and diacylglycerol lipase-β (DAGLβ). The metabolizing enzymes are fatty acid amide hydrolase (FAAH) and monoacylglycerol lipase (MGL).

may actually inhibit the activity of the proteins. We mostly want these receptors being active and activated! Since the book is about the ECS it will mainly focus on the effects of THC on systems and will cover cannabinoids occurring in other plants too that can benefit our ECS function. Plants are complex mixtures of hundreds of compounds that traditionally have been considered to work synergistically and this is true for cannabis. In addition to the cannabinoid class of compounds there are terpenoids, amino acids, fatty acids, sterols, esters, flavonoids and more! This work will focus mostly on what is know about the major active ingredients: cannabinoids and terpenoids.

> **HERBAN LEGEND 1:** CBD activates CB2 and THC activates CB1. CBD does not appear to either directly, or indirectly, modulate the ECS. Marketing messages around CBD claim that it will boost levels of AEA, indirectly affecting the ECS. Research has not yet widely substantiated this claim. Therefore, I primarily refer to THC as the cannabis phytochemical that is the primary activator of the ECS.

Like many other of our biological systems (cardiovascular, metabolic, musculoskeletal), the ECS exhibits activity that varies across the human lifespan with peak function occurring in adolescence and early adulthood. Since the ECS can be modulated using pharmacy (either plant or synthetic chemicals) it makes sense that health status and age would affect to what extent the system may *need* to be modulated. This translates to: dosing for THC is not one-size-fits-all, the way that most pharmaceutical therapies are used.

The ECS is the template or construct we will use to walk through our system's biology. Systems biology is a means to help understand the big picture. In present-day medicine, each of our systems has been given over to specialists and we have a cardiologist and nephrologist and a neurologist and a hepatologist and a gynecologist- different doctors for different systems. It is often necessary to get more of a bird's-eye view of how all of the pieces (systems) operate together to inform health, rather than taking a reductionist approach by examining the pieces separately. The ECS in every tissue in the human body is one that can tie all the other systems together. It is an efficient system that can easily be modulated and return quickly to baseline. By its nature, the ECS demonstrates what resilience is! It is known to be involved in the initiation and termination of our nervous response to stress, regulation of appetite, fat storage, sleep, immunity, storing memory, and reproduction. These are some of the reasons why it is known as our global, homeostatic modulatory system.

Some important terminology to keep in mind:

- **Homeostasis** is the means by which an organism reaches and maintains its *stable optimum setpoint* (similarly to how an air conditioner keeps the room air at a certain temperature). This concept can be applied across tissues—and multidimensionally—to tell the physiologic response story. There are a host of chemical messengers that act as positive and negative feedback signals in loops. All of our organs and systems participate in this process, and the ECS is our body's thermostat. It's a relay, a cross-talker, a language that every system has to speak similar to the operating system on a computer.

  Physician and author Gabor Maté said, "To say that the nervous system is connected to the immune system, and the immune system is connected to the emotional apparatus, all of which is connected to the hormone system, is incorrect. They are not connected; they are the same system."[5] What makes them the same is the ECS, the operating system that knows all other systems' code.

- **Hormesis** is a characteristic of many biological processes, describing the conditions that shape how we adapt to environmental perturbations (either slight or extreme). These adaptations result in alterations of our biochemical messaging. As humans, we must adapt in order to survive. For example, a small dose of mercury could be beneficial for stimulating our detoxification pathways, but a large or even moderate dose over a long period of time can also be toxic—damaging to cells and tissues. Low amounts may produce the opposite effects from high amounts. This hormetic concept can be applied to the ECS and to dosing of THC. Reducing levels of ECS functioning may be needed in some situations while increasing the level of function are needed in other settings. Somewhere in the middle, where we probably want to be, is tone. Tone means that we are strong, resilient, and efficient. Learning when and how to balance, whether to stimulate or suppress, can be a delicate affair. Both CB1R and CB2R mediate hormetic responses, which can occur either in the short or long term. I refer to this as tone (low dose THC), hack (moderate dose THC), or suppress (high dose THC).

- **Allostasis** was originally considered to be an expansion of homeostasis. Allostasis is now considered to be stability through change, a subtype of homeostasis. This process becomes important in the setting of chronic stress, or repeated ups and downs. Think of this like wear and tear in this case on your tissues and organs. In the long term, the body/mind adaptations to stress have been defined as allostatic load.[6]

- *Allostatic load (AL)* is the cost of chronic exposure to stress. Stress results in fluctuating or increased bodily responses that come from repeated or chronic environmental challenges we react to as stressful. The strain on the body produced by repeated ups and downs and the associated bodily responses, the elevated activity of physiologic systems under challenge, is taxing. This culminates in a predisposition to disease (either a literal disease or a state of lacking ease). Increased AL, which can be measured using laboratory testing, is associated with a large variety of physiological problems. These include obesity, metabolic syndrome, hypertension, hyperlipidemia, inflammation, atherosclerosis, ulcers, and cardiovascular disorders. The overarching goal of this book is to reduce your AL.

- **Resilience** is the ability to adapt to and spring back from difficulty or hard times. Our body's chemistry is modified in the short and long term by negative experiences. Resilience includes the ability to rebound from physical, emotional, mental, and biochemical stressors. Some of these adaptations require emotional and behavioral skills that don't come naturally to us or that we were not formally taught. Our body's systems control and determine our responses.

The ECS has been called a construct- a concept or a model. From basic science we know that cell stress leads to ECB release and the concentration of these compounds determines either cell survival or cell death. Important stressful events inside the cell determine our homeostasis or allostasis. This is why the ECS master regulatory system needs to be well-toned in order to bring systems homeostasis. The original, intended setpoints (the default setting) are the most efficient for survival. Consider this to be like energy efficiency. The ability to consciously modify responses to stress, to cultivate and practice skills that enhance stress resilience, and to tone the ECS are all imperative for helping you harness your energy, protect cells and promote health and wellbeing.

- Step 1: Acknowledge stressors and their impacts on the body/mind.
- Step 2: Begin to adjust your lifestyle and treat your biochemistry, tone the ECS.
- Step 3: Hack the ECS when indicated but only temporarily while you work on treating the whole person rather than symptoms.

By addressing the whole person and building strong foundations of health you can stop, and potentially reverse, the destructive impacts of chronic stress on your life. In this book you will learn to use the ECS as a template for a step-by-step approach to help restore your ability to respond to stress positively so that all of your systems are on go.

Appetite and metabolism (eat), sleeping (sleep), anxiety/fear (relax), immune function (protect), and memory (forget) are automatic (or autonomic) functions our body needs to be able to respond to input from the environment and from our internal sensors and to survive. We don't think about having these responses generally, as they are primal and basic to our survival.

Nearly 50 years after THC was first isolated and subsequently led to the discovery of the ECS (starting in the 1990s) much more is known about how the ECS has been conserved across evolutionary time. This conservation allows mammals to overcome the consequences of stress and to achieve recovery as efficiently as possible. As the science of the ECS has progressed, these interactions are proving to be not as simple as initially thought. This book seeks to simplify and inform about the innerworkings of this system to illustrate how necessary a well-functioning ECS is for resilience and health. Surviving *and* thriving are the topics of this book.

Adversity can come in many forms. There is a myriad of resources for you to explore (starting with adverse childhood experiences [ACEs]) to tally the hallmarks from childhood that may have affected your biochemistry and contributed to health risk factors.[7] Don't discount that there may have been trauma in your life given that no remembered event is *too small* to be counted as adverse. In fact, it is not necessarily the event, or the magnitude of the traumatic event that matters, but rather your unique responses and adaptations made around these events that are at the heart of the matter.

Meeting with a qualified psychologist/therapist who is trauma-informed is an important tool to help move through and past these events. Using psychological and behavioral tools can help you identify your past adaptations and how these may now be maladaptive. Therapy is one of several integral pieces that will put you on the path to restoring your health.

The broad systemic effects of trauma include:

- Cardiovascular: Blood pressure, cardiovascular disease, clotting disorders, stroke
- Mental health: Post-traumatic stress disorder (PTSD), poor stress resilience, chronic anxiety, depression, bipolar depression
- Immune system: Suppression, inflammation, increased susceptibility to illness, including autoimmune and cancer
- Genitourinary system: Chronic pelvic pain, bladder infections, vaginal pain,
- Musculoskeletal system: Fibromyalgia, fatigue, joint pain, low back pain, chronic pain
- Endocrine: Diabetes risk, thyroid problems, reproductive problems (infertility, endometriosis, menstrual pain)

- Neurological: Memory impairment, risk of dementia, neurological diseases, neuropathic pain

How does the ECS play a role in the stress response and recovery from impaired stress resilience? This is an elaborate story that this book will unpack for you. You need to be intimate with the ECS to be able to use it as your guide. Clinical studies show that endocannabinoids are a barometer for stress and that stress-related disorders impact ECS homeostasis.

Chronic stress suppresses the production of AEA, our body's bliss molecule. Chronic stress also impairs the ability of AEA to activate CB1R due to downregulation of the protein (amount of the protein receptor is reduced). This process uncouples the system from efficiently performing its natural role of homeostasis, and also the body's ability to reach allostasis. With long-term stress, 2AG production goes up. We register stress first in the body, then in the mind.

ECBs are closely associated with the stress response and related inflammation. They also appear to play an important role in the brain by promoting forgetting. A part of our brain performs something called extinction learning. If our brains remembered every single detail of each moment, we would overload. In short, forgetting entails a gradual decrease in our response to a conditioned stimulus. For example, any personal danger trigger you can identify that causes you to startle, increases your heart rate, gives you dry mouth, sweat, feeling dizzy or shaky. This response is automatic (our autonomic nervous system)—the fight-or-flight response, or adrenaline rush. The endocannabinoid system is suggested as a prime target for treating this type of anxiety in general, and for post-traumatic stress disorder (PTSD) in particular.

Cannabinoids and cannabis compounds (at therapeutic doses) have a relationship to AL due to their beneficial effects on stress. This includes both their ability to aid in forgetting bad memories, and their anti-inflammatory potential. Inflammation markers are a component of AL (such as cortisol and other inflammatory compounds). Our natural ECBs are the messengers by which we return to our desired setpoint—internal peace and the associated physiology, biochemistry. This is what we need for our optimal physical, mental, and emotional health—survival. Achieving stability through change is the literal physical process on which our survival relies, and is the adventure you have embarked upon by engaging with this book.

If the stress response is sub-optimal (for any reason) the ECS may need a push from our plant allies! Plants have moved civilizations for millennia (think of spices, caffeine and sugar) and cannabinoids may be calling you to facilitate your personal health evolution. You can transform with or without using cannabis because there are also dietary cannabinoids and activities to engage in that can help to tone your ECS.

Stress is a major health problem costing more than $300 billion a year and shortening life expectancy. With stress in modern society continuing to rise, we need a method to reverse the negative health impacts. The terroir (from French- a term that describes your environment) of this book will allow you to map how you are shaped by what is around you! This is a walk that invites the *whole person* to participate: the body *and* mind. There will be elements that will focus on activities such as food, pleasure, contemplation, becoming intimate with others, modifying your relationship with sleep, relaxing, playing, and forgetting. Don't forget that the construct for describing what the ECS does for us is to provide that we "eat, sleep, relax, protect, and forget." We will delve into each of these areas, and you will chart a course for how you can tap into the majesty of this system to help you increase your resilience to stress, to heal, and to live a healthy life.

You have probably heard of mind/body medicine, a paradigm-shifting approach in patient care that connects how we think with how we feel and our general well-being. I focus on body/mind* medicine—the chemical mediators, both endo-chemicals and plant-based chemicals, that can promote resilience, restore homeostasis and reverse the AL that suppresses healing. Within this body/mind approach, the interface is the immune system and transmitters that are shared between the body and brain. The body has its

---

* Candace Pert was an internationally known neurobiologist (discoverer of the opioid receptor) who said "the body and mind are not separate and we cannot treat one without the other".

own brain that you can learn to tune into. Then, using plant allies, we can tap into the healing power of nature and the ECS. Toning the ECS will help you to restore, revive, and recover from generations of trauma-induced biochemical impairments to survivability!

There are 5 chapters in the book: Eat, Sleep, Relax, Protect, and Forget. Each chapter is organized with an overview of the topic, and then a deep dive:

- How the ECS functions within each system
- Background on cannabis for system function
- Body/mind activity: improving interoception
- Case in point: a patient case for illustration
- Women's health related to system function
- Disorders related to function of the system
- Naturopathic/Integrative/Functional Approaches for systems toning
  - Toning the ECS
  - Terpenes
  - Measuring AL
  - Herbal allies
  - Supplements
  - Things to avoid
  - Food/nutritional approaches
  - Chakras and yoga

Yoga is integral for toning the ECS. Understanding how yoga works and why it is important will assist you. While yoga has its roots in Hinduism, it has been widely used as a tool to work with the energy in the body through the science of pranayama, or energy control. Yoga comes from the root word in Sanskrit that can be translated to mean "unite" or yoking of the body and mind. Prana is from the Sanskrit word translated to mean "life force" or "vital principle". Chakra comes from the Sanskrit word meaning "wheel". Chakras are focal points or nodes along our spine, from the coccyx to the top of the head. Awakening and energizing chakras are practices found in traditions beyond Hinduism. One chakra will be highlighted for each chapter of the book and the sixth introduced here. There are a number of types of yoga practices, but here I focus on the asanas, or physical postures, and breathwork called pranayama. Both practices have known health benefits and are intended to help to balance energy in the body.

> *"The higher teachings of yoga take one beyond techniques, and show the yogi, or yoga practitioner, how to direct his concentration in such a way as not only to harmonize human with divine consciousness, but to merge his consciousness in the Infinite."*
> —Paramahansa Yogananda, father of Western yoga

Yoga teaches how to still the mind through breath control and to attain higher states of awareness. A yoga practice can help to improve our interoception.*

Anahata Chakra

I'll start with the fourth chakra, Anahata, which means unstuck, which is hopefully what this book will help address: stuckness. The color associated with Anahata is green. This chakra is anatomically associated with the center of the chest or sternum, where the cardiac plexus of nerves is. It is often called the heart chakra or the energetic hub of our emotions. Stress, bad memories, overthinking and emotional pain can block this chakra. Expanding the chest, pulling the shoulders back and lifting the heart to the sky is one way to open this energy center. This pose also increases circulation to the heart and lungs. This opening posture is reputed to enhance the quality of our love and our experience of peace. Means of stabilizing this chakra include practicing self-compassion which can lead to empathy for others; practicing gratitude; practicing receiving gifts; and asking for help

---

* Our brain is constantly tracking internal signals to optimize function across the body. Being conscious of what is happening in our body is called interoception-the process of sensing signals from the body. One way to check in on your interoception is to sit still and see how good you are at feeling your heart beat. If you have a wearable device that counts your heart rate, use this monitor to compare how many beats you can count in a minute to the monitor's count. You can also ask someone else to count your pulse for a minute while you also count. Emotional events that we experience often start somewhere in our body. Learning to become attuned to these signals improves self-regulation.

or helping others. These concepts are related to our well-being as self-acceptance is essential for healing.

- Asanas for this chakra include dhanurasana (bow pose), ustrasana (camel), urdhva dhanurasana (bridge or wheel), and virabhadrasana II (warrior pose).
- Pranayama bhramari is for the heart. Often called humming bee's breath, bhramari is thought to be healing for the anahata chakra. Place your thumbs on the outer ears to shut out sound. Place your other fingers along the skull like a cradle for your head. Slowly inhale through your nose and hum for the entire exhalation so that air slowly leaves your lungs with a soft sound, at a pitch that is comfortable for your throat. You should be able to feel vibrations in your chest. Start with a few rounds and the add more over time, up to 10 breaths. This should leave you feeling calm, more in control of your emotions, less stressed, and may help to reduce blood pressure.

For some, cannabis can be an aid to athletic performance and exercise can boost the ECS. One small study in people with coronary artery disease found that smoking cannabis decreased the time to exhaustion, suggesting improved endurance while another study found the opposite.[8, 9] However, cannabis can also elevate heart rate which could be dangerous for some, especially with unstable heart disease. Due to CB1R located in and around blood vessels, a rapid effect of inhaled cannabis is dilation of blood vessels (vasodilation). This can lead to a precipitous drop in blood pressure and increased delivery of blood (and oxygen) to tissues. The transient drop in blood pressure for those with low blood pressure can lead to orthostatic hypotension where blood moves rapidly to the legs upon standing. This can cause dizziness, lightheadedness, and an elevation of the heart rate in an effort to pump blood back up to the brain. This effect may be increased by physical activity or being over-heated. Those with low blood pressure need to exercise caution. THC also induces opening of the airways (bronchioles) and this may be another way that cannabis could influence athletic performance. Given the increase in circulation and delivery of oxygen to the tissues, cannabis can be a potentially good companion for yoga. THC may act on the stretch reflex and therefore be an aid for improving flexibility.[10]

Conversely, exercise boosts ECS function. There have been a number of studies in humans and animals showing that exercise increases the levels of ECBs in the blood.[11, 12] Moderate intensity exercise is apparently the optimal level for boosting ECB levels.[13] ECBs are partially responsible for the "runner's high' and this knowledge serves to support that boosting ECS function can bring the rewards of well-being, euphoria and reduced anxiety without even using cannabis![14]

It is time to jump into this journey with an intention to become unstuck. Remember that this is a traveling, a slow going from one place to another, as if on a slow boat, a slow walk or a slow-moving train. Think of it as akin to swimming upstream, which can feel like slow progress and hard work, but the end result being that of altering your life's trajectory!

Through a collaboration with the software company OnTracka, the creator Chad Walkaden has generously provided you access to a smart phone application to track your progress as you move through this book. This book/app collaboration is intended to provide you with a technology that allows real-time, secure tracking to manage your health, keep calm, track dosing, and monitor other aspects of your lifestyle. Watch for the QR code located throughout the book for opportunities to engage!

Please consider signing up for Dr. Sexton's newsletter by going to ecsdoctor.com. This email list will update you on news related to the book, speaking tours, give-aways and for opportunities to try out new products and participate in market research using OnTracka!

Access supplements that are known and trusted through Fullscript. Look for a protocol for each chapter in your account.

Access trusted hemp cannabinoid products at Myriam's Hemp.

CHAPTER 1:

Eat

Overview

Our relationship with food is complex and multilayered. Food is necessary for survival. Eating is comforting. Food provides us with nutrients. Eating is a social experience. For some, the feeling of hunger can be distressing and for others hunger is a satisfying feeling of emptiness. Our relationship with hunger is part of instinctive survival. How we experience hunger can provide clues about our body/mind, our ability to interpret our body signals, and help to understand our rate of metabolism—the chemical process of making energy. You, or someone you know, may be hypervigilant for hunger or have a quick metabolism. These people may frequently feel hungry or worried about their next meal, both of which are emotional aspects of our relationship with food. Alternatively, fasting can be easy for some and difficult or impossible for others. How are food, eating, and metabolism related to the ECS?

From the womb, we are endowed with a natural reflex for sucking in preparation for our first encounter with food, previously provided by the placenta. In a famous study performed in neonatal mice (the first few days of life) by Israeli scientist Esther Fride in 2002, blockade of the CB1 receptor (CB1R) by a drug given intravenously (IV) demonstrated the importance of the ECS in the suckling reflex.

In these CB1-blocked mice, their growth was halted and, further, led to the death of the animals. The cause of death was an oral motor defect, the result of blocking the receptor. The oral motor defect means that the mice lost their sucking reflex; they could not eat to survive. This experiment shows how the ECS from the beginning of life outside the womb is paramount for our survival.[15]

Newborn mothers are vigilant when their babies appear to be failing to thrive—a condition where babies are not gaining weight or length at a normal rate. It has been suggested that deficiencies or dysfunction of the ECS, such as with the CB1R may be an underlying cause of non-organic failure to thrive, no known reason why growth slowed. Breast milk is rich in endocannabinoid compounds, which is likely one reason why babies appear drunk when they finish breastfeeding. However, breast milk cannabinoids are not the same as the ECBs.

> **HERBAN LEGEND #2:** Because ECBs are in breast milk, cannabis and THC is safe for babies. This is not a rational assumption. THC is a much more potent molecule and the resulting effects will not be identical to ECBs binding CBRs. There is more about cannabis and human development in pregnancy in the chapter Relax.

We need to be able to accurately interpret our hunger signals. Interoception is an innate function that can sometimes be deficient due to exposures when the brain is forming. Emotional exposures or inborn genetics, in particular, can have effects on our interoceptive abilities. Throughout this book you will rate your interoceptive abilities using a tool that is also useful for toning the ECS—a Scale of Body Connection.[16] Here is your initial assessment. This is a tool we will come back to and monitor how you are doing with improving your stress resilience over time.

Based on your self-evaluation, place yourself on a continuum by marking the line where you believe you fall between the 2 extremes of body awareness and body detachment. Do you perceive yourself more toward body aware or at the other end, as extremely detached from your body? Or do you fall somewhere in between? Rate yourself for your awareness or detachment from your body.

Body Connection Assessment:

First place yourself on the line.

←――――――――――――――――――――――――――→

++Body Awareness **Body Detachment++**

Make a list of 3 things you think you may be detached from in your body.

1. _____

2. _____

3. _____

Now make a list of 3 things you feel most connected to in your body.

1. _____

2. _____

3. _____

This scale represents your sensitivity to signals in your body and provides one measure of interoception, a somewhat hidden sense that underlies our well-being. This is a concept that I aim to help you develop using the ECS as a guide. You can become expert at knowing what you are feeling and understanding what is going on inside of your body. By listening and responding to our body's intelligence, we can promote physical, mental, emotional, and spiritual health.

The ECS Provides That We Eat

The ECS is known to regulate appetite, food intake, energy production (metabolism), digestion, gut motility, and intestinal inflammation. The ECS also interacts with the many bacteria that live in our gastrointestinal tracts (the microbiome).

One of the best known roles for CB1R is orexia: stimulating the desire for food, appetite, increasing food desirability, and promoting eating behavior. Disruptions to the ECS have been associated with disordered eating (restrictive, compulsive, or inflexible eating patterns), metabolic disruptions (diabetes/obesity/wasting syndrome), and gastrointestinal motility problems (nausea, constipation, diarrhea, or gastroparesis). These conditions are an indication that the ECS is not functioning optimally. Because the ECS is found in the brain and in the gastrointestinal (GI) system (and everywhere in between) it is a common thread uniting the body/mind. It relays communication between nerves, tissues (such as muscle cells and glands that secrete hormones and enzymes into the GI tract) and between systems (as between the nervous and GI systems).

Our ECBs (body-made cannabinoids) are manufactured from fatty acids that we get from our diet. (See Box 1.2.) The 2 primary ECBs, considered primary because they are a part of families of compounds, directly activate the CBR1 and CBR2: AEA (arachidonylethanolamine or anandamide) and 2AG (2-arachidonylglycerol). Made from arachidonic acid (an omega-6 fatty acid), found across many foods, both plant- and animal-based. (The family of ECBs are made from other fatty acid chains.) The CB1R is found in the brain, on and in nerve cells, fat cells, skeletal muscle, liver tissue, (spread ubiquitously across every tissue in the body)—all of these tissues are involved in eating and metabolism. Metabolism is the chemical process of converting food to energy (the basic human energy unit is adenosine triphosphate [ATP]), to help us grow, be healthy, reproduce, and store energy for future use as fat. ECBs even have a rhythm—the highest amount of 2AG measured in blood occurs at midday and has been associated with the time of day that our ancestors were hunting and foraging.

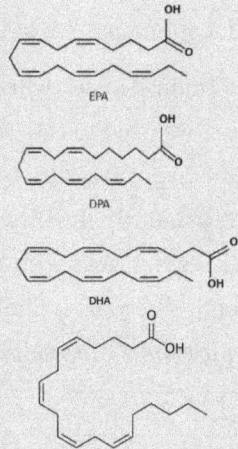

BOX 1.2 FATTY ACIDS

Omega 3 fatty acids: Anti-inflammatory and critical to health. Our body does not make them so we have to get them from dietary sources.

Arachidonic acid (AA): ECBs are made from this! Generally, AA contributes to inflammation as it dominates our diet, found in both plant and animal-based foods.

The lines represent carbons and carbon bonds. Fatty acids are carbon chains of different lengths with an 'acid' on the end.

Research strongly suggests that the ECS plays an important role in our survival by stimulating hunger, enhancing our desire for food, and regulating our expenditure of calories. The ECS controls food intake through specific structures in the brain, including the hypothalamus, a major hub involved as a relay station in the regulation of body temperature, emotional responses, and feeding and energy balance. (Elsewhere, its role in sleep regulation, the stress response, reproduction, immune sensing, learning and memory and aging is discussed.)

The hypothalamus-gut-axis (HGA) or, more commonly, the gut-brain axis, is a two-way street, where the enteric nervous system, a specialized nervous system in the gut, the microbiome, and specialized immune tissue in the gut are all communicating with the brain.

The hypothalamus is a collection of neurons in the brain and is the hub for hunger control. Interestingly, it is also closely associated with brain regions that control our emotions, pain perception, growth, stress, and fear. CB1R in this area of the brain have been shown to regulate our literal energetic balance.[17] The network of communications with the hypothalamus helps explain why there are so many things we experience that can affect hunger. Human survival depends on the ability to eat, to store excess energy (fat), and to meet energy demands when food is scarce. Eating behavior is controlled by homeostatic processes; orexigenic* describes signaling that induces hunger. We have to be hungry to survive.

The brain decides whether we have the energy stores we need to survive and if we need to eat. The ECS stimulates us to eat. When ECB levels go up in the hypothalamus, binding to the CB1R leads to the desire to eat.[18] This rise, primarily in AEA, activates the reward center in the brain, a process that is associated with the release of the neurotransmitter dopamine. This chemical reward is one way that eating, or being satiated after eating, gives us pleasure. Other sensory signals such as sight and smell contribute to the orexic effects.

AEA has a functional relationship with two other eating-related chemicals: leptin and gastrin. Gastrin is made in the stomach and its release as a chemical messenger triggers the hypothalamus to induce hunger. On the other hand, leptin made in fat cells resolves hunger by acting as a chemical messenger in the same part of the brain. Once our hunger is satiated, leptin levels go up, gastrin levels go down. AEA returns to its former level and we are at homeostasis.

If our body does not have enough energy, we will feel physical hunger, which can be uncomfortable or interpreted as a painful sensation by some people—a cue that energy reserves may be low. These feelings, for people who may have experienced food insecurity, are undesirable sensations. Getting hangry (acting angry when actually hungry) is a form of hunger that is emotional and can reflect a physical detachment from the body. Some people can have low blood sugar and have dizziness, shakiness, anxiety, irritability, and sweating. Recognizing hunger is an aspect of interoception, and a sense that can be learned with practice. Emotional hunger, eating for emotional comfort when feeling emotionally empty, is something that may have been programmed into your brain as a child.

Cannabis has been used as an appetite regulator from ancient times.[19] Cannabis activates the ECS by THC binding to CBRs. THC is considered a partial agonist at CBRs, but has and affinity (ease of forming a chemical bond)

---

* From the Greek orexic, meaning hunger and genic, to stimulate.

for the receptors higher than that of our ECBs. (See Box 1.3.) Cannabis is well-known for causing the munchies. Munchies, or hedonic eating, are a sudden surge in appetite and desire for certain foods after using cannabis. This is a drive to eat for pleasure, even when calories are not needed. This can be a great benefit for some (such as those undergoing cancer therapies) and perhaps a pitfall for others! You can measure your hedonic hunger before and after cannabis use using a power of food scale.[20, 21]

BOX 1.3   PHARMACOLOGY TERMS

AGONIST: A chemical that can bind to and activate a receptor. Binding triggers a response that may mimic that of a naturally occurring substance. An agonist be classified as full, partial, or inverse agonist.

ANTAGONIST: A chemical that does not produce a biological response on binding to a receptor. Instead, the binding blocks or reduces the effect of an agonist. The binding may be competitive or non-competitive (binds to the same place or not).

POTENCY OR AFFINITY: A way to measure the effective concentration (dose) of a drug. Affinity depends on the nature of the ligand and the receptor.

LIGAND: A molecule that binds to another molecule.

BINDING: The act of chemical attraction where forces bring a small molecule or protein together with another, leading to a reaction.

The CB1R plays a role in our sensory perception of food by both taste and smell (more associated 2AG signaling in this case)! There are CB1Rs on your tastebuds, thought to enhance sweet taste reception![22] Higher 2AG levels in the blood have been associated with higher food intake, while blocking the CB1R inhibits appetite.[23] It is important to note that there are minimal studies or research in humans outside of helping with appetite in people with HIV/AIDs or undergoing cancer therapy. Most of the data is from research conducted on animals. In short, the ECS plays a clear role in eating behavior, keeping our metabolic balance in homeostasis by promoting hunger, and is specifically designed to favor the accumulation of energy![24] Unfortunately, this can lead to eating too many calories and storing more fat for some people.

Green Energy

We have a built-in chemical and physiological ability to be resilient to stress. We also have a form of built-in metabolic resilience or flexibility. Metabolic flexibility is the ability to adapt our energy demand in response to available fuel or vice versa. Flexibility in the dynamics around our energy is programmed by the inherited genes from our biological parents (genetics) as well as what we are exposed to in the environment. There are environmental effects (prevailing conditions) including our activity levels, and effects on us or our ancestors such as food availability, trauma, toxic stress, and pollution (chemical exposures). Metabolic flexibility is central to evolution and survival, as those who can subsist for the longest and adapt to changing conditions, or make it on the least amount of food, will survive! Changes resulting from these external conditions determine how (which and how much) our genes are expressed and this is called epigenetics.

Have you ever tried fasting (going without food) or subsisting only on water for any amount of time? Some will say they absolutely cannot do it, while others may find it relatively easy to do. I have been able to fast for up to 14 days with no ill effects, other than the first 2–3 days of feeling hungry. This is an example of metabolic flexibility- easily adapting to changes in metabolic/energy demands and/or food availability; it is a form of physiologic adaptability.

Our bodies need to be able to switch fuel burning capability (such as from protein, fat, or carbohydrate fuel sources) to burning ketone bodies (what we burn when fasting) to storage of fuel as glycogen or fat to burn later. The amount of fuel we burn, as during exercise, is dictated by our skeletal muscle, fat stores, and energy exchanges going across the networks between tissues. The macronutrients we eat (fat, protein, sugars) have shifted and changed over generations; humans have needed to be able to shift and change the storage and use of currently available energy.

The process of energy production is complex and wondrous! I was surprised when I took one of my first chemistry classes to learn that oxygen (which we need to survive) is also responsible for harm to the body. All of our energy storage/ use is ultimately regulated by tiny cell inclusions, mitochondria, that every cell in our body contains. This power supply, which is like a battery or power source at the level of individual cells, has the CB1R!

The CB1R at the level of mitochondria is not yet completely understood, but is known to be involved in regulating the manufacture of adenosine triphosphate (ATP), the basic energy unit at the cellular level (the respiratory chain). In the process of this ATP-making, known as mitochondrial respiration, reactive oxygen species (ROS) are an inevitable byproduct. When reactive oxygen is formed, it can wreak havoc on tissues by causing damage to proteins, lipids (fats), and even our DNA. Whenever ROS are produced, the ECS is there to provide homeostasis for the redox reactions—the process by which ROS can be tamed (reduced) by our body systems. We need balance between generating reactive oxygen and quenching it. A little bit of stress can tone us while too much will break us down. CB1R binding induces an enzyme, nitric oxide synthase (iNOS), which slows down the mitochondrial activity, and can either reduce or promote the production of reactive oxygen species (ROS). We need optimal function of our ECS to produce energy and to balance the good vs. evil in the production of our molecular fuel. This is another homeostatic role of the ECS.

You are made of over 37 trillion cells, *not* counting the bacteria that we co-exist with, thought to number close to a quintillion cells. We share mitochondria with bacterial ancestors, as they are the source from which mitochondria evolved (archaebacteria). These forms of life likely also manufactured ECBs.[25] The co-evolution of life and ECS appear to go hand-in-hand. Further mind-blowing is the fact that every cell in our body can contain from 200 to 10,000 mitochondria! The mitochondrial CB1R is described as controlling energy production at this very basic level. The ECS is ancient, going back to the time of early evolution, and plays essential roles in basic survival through energy production and adaptation to energy sources.

To Eat or Not to Eat

Signaling through CB1R is an efficient means to adjust metabolism for energy storage for future energy needs. The outcomes of this signaling include eating more, desiring energy-rich food, increasing insulin secretion from the pancreas, moderating the use of glucose by skeletal muscles and regulating digestion—from breakdown of food to uptake of nutrients and distributing fat. During digestion, ECS signaling is involved in exocrine functions of the GI (glands that release products),* as the ECS is monitoring and gating the release of pancreatic enzymes. In addition, insulin secretion, necessary for utilization of glucose (what our body makes from all carbohydrates) is regulated by the ECS, implicating targeting this system to treat diabetes.[26] In a nutshell, all of these things are related to survival by supporting resilience in the face of danger and to help us be ready to engage in a search for fuel.

If it were possible to block the CB1 receptor, what would happen? This approach was tried as a means to treat obesity with a drug called rimonabant™ in 2007, an antagonist at the CB1R for inducing anorexia (the opposite of orexia- a lack of appetite).[27] Unfortunately, this antagonism of the CB1R came with unwanted side effects of depression, anxiety, and suicidal thoughts and the drug was withdrawn due to these side effects. Treatment with this drug had some success in reducing obesity however, this CB1R blockade was not such a good idea due to the role in mood regulation. The CB2R has also been reported to be involved in energy homeostasis, although through anti-inflammatory mechanisms, as this protein is primarily associated with immune cells and tissues. Strategies targeting the CB2R are being investigated for potential anti-obesity effects. (Find more information in Chapter Protect.) There is a pharmaceutical company that has developed a CB1R antibody (another way of blocking the receptor) to treat non-alcoholic liver disease. Do you wonder if this is a good idea, given the broad role for CB1R signaling across many systems and the role in providing us with bliss?

Paradoxically, ECS signaling also increases in the setting of overnutrition, which ultimately can result in obesity and type 2 diabetes. Both of these

---

* Exocrine relates to glands that secrete substances such as sweat, tears, saliva, milk, and digestive juices. Endocrine refers to glands that secrete substances (hormones) into the blood stream to travel around the body and serve as messengers for metabolism, growth, and reproduction.

two are conditions of being overfed and are pro-inflammatory, implicating a role for the CB2R. When we are fed, the hormone leptin is a reflection of this state, as our fat cells primarily secrete this compound when fatty acid accumulation has occurred. Release of leptin is under the control of the CB1R in fat cells and leptin release reduces CB1R expression in the hypothalamus (a brain area that links our endocrine system with the nervous system).[28] This ever-fluctuating signaler feeds back to the hypothalamus to communicate "no more food needed" thereby inducing anorexia or turning down the volume on appetite.

During lean times, such as fasting or not eating for several hours, leptin levels go down and this messages the hypothalamus: hunger! In part, this happens by increasing AEA signaling at CB1R in the hypothalamus. Leptin is more involved in energy control over the long-term than meal-to-meal and also involved in maintaining optimal weight. THC acting at CB1R can stimulate appetite whether or not you may have eaten recently, so it overrides the system. Great for when you need a hack, (like during cancer treatments) but it can be undesirable when you are well- or overfed.

Obesity is a global problem, and in the US over 35% of people, mainly women, are affected. The direct cause is excess of calories; for women, hormones and insulin resistance due to malfunctioning hormones are also contributors. The ECS shifts our energy balance toward storing of energy and promotion of fat storage. If it were possible to limit the CB1 blockade only to fat cells, this could be an approach way to improve metabolism and bypass the brain effects that led to depression in the clinical trial of CB1R blockade.

The opposite of the fed state, food deprivation, is intertwined with a more famous, meal-to-meal hormone made in the stomach: grehlin. When grehlin is secreted in the stomach, it activates the ECS by increasing AEA production in the hypothalamus. This AEA binds to the CB1R, sends the signal up the vagus nerve to the brainstem and stimulates appetite. Fasting has also been associated with inducing AEA, so it appears that this ECB is working alongside grehlin to produce the feeling of hunger and to stimulate appetite.

Grehlin is also interesting because other brain targets are the pituitary gland (just below the hypothalamus). Picture this gland it like the brain's testicles (sitting in a protected place, by the way). There are two lobes and each produces different chemical messengers. Pituitary releases growth hormones, the GI muscles start moving, and the pancreas secretes insulin to move glucose into cells. Grehlin is in the driver's seat for a lot of things. In some cases, the desire is to increase grehlin levels (as in irritable bowel syndrome or gastritis) but decrease the levels in others (anorexia, irritable bowel disease). The ECS is the mediator between the two extremes of grehlin amount, and by toning the ECS it is possible to modulate both hunger and biochemistry beneficially, skewing toward survival.

Different Effects of Cannabinoids at Different Doses

An interesting concept is that ECBs and PCBs have both been shown to have biphasic effects. This literally means two phases, for example low doses could be stimulating while high doses sedative. Or low dose reduces anxiety and high dose induces anxiety. Different doses can induce different or even opposite effects. To complicate this more, the same dose given to a young person vs. an older person may lead to different effects, another form of being biphasic, based on age.[29] This concept is also known as hormesis and represents a form of biological plasticity,* where low-level (low dose) stimulation can be beneficial (this is true even for stress) and high-level (or high dose) stimulation can be toxic. This applies to many compounds, whether made in the body, by plants, or in a laboratory.

As an example, low-dose THC, which activates the CB1R, will most likely induce hunger (orexia), while high-dose THC, over time, can induce anorexia (lack of hunger). At a high dose, THC will start binding other off-target proteins and the ECS can also be suppressed. The body compensates for excessive receptor activation, either by a single high dose and by chronic high doses of THC, by turning off receptors or decreasing their number and depleting our supply of ECBs.

---

* Plasticity is a primary feature of the human body that allows continuously for acquiring and maintaining function. This process is at the heart of adaptability to our environments.

A meta-analysis of cannabis users vs. non-users found that the body mass index (BMI) of cannabis users was lower that than of non-users.[30] Could this be an example of suppression? THC can either augment or inhibit neurotransmission by activating or blocking receptors, depending on the dose or use over time. (See Figure 1.1.)

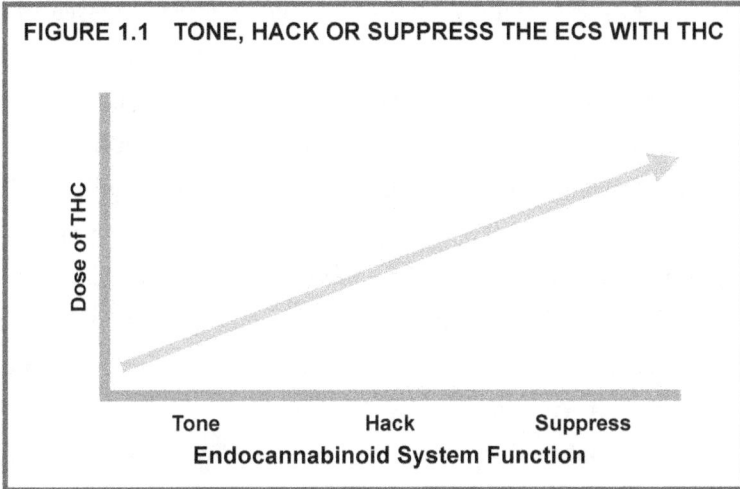

FIGURE 1.1 TONE, HACK OR SUPPRESS THE ECS WITH THC

Dose of THC

Tone   Hack   Suppress
Endocannabinoid System Function

Downregulation of CB1R, or a reduction in the amount of receptor, is associated with high THC potency cannabis: dabbing, using waxes and concentrates, and chronic daily heavy use of cannabis. In summary, a very low dose is more likely to tone the ECS, a moderate dose is a hack for the system, and a high dose will suppress ECS function.

In persons who are overweight (defined medically as having a BMI of >30), the ECS is dysregulated in fat tissues, where ECB levels are high. This high concentration acts locally to downregulate the CB1R. When the receptor is downregulated, the receptor activation by an agonist (THC, AEA or 2AG) could be likened to giving a high dose (there are fewer receptors and this increases sensitivity of the receptor), not thought to be beneficial for health. What happens in this context is an increase in making of new fat cells (lipogenesis), which leads to compounding weight gain. This appears to happen by downregulation of the enzyme that breaks down AEA, FAAH. This results in increasing the levels of AEA locally (less FAAH = more AEA). If we could measure ECBs in the blood easily, it is unclear what these levels would reveal about this scenario because the ECS is finely tuned in each tissue compartment, locally, and not necessarily reflected by what we would measure in the blood.

For example, 2AG levels have been found to be elevated in circulating levels (blood) of people with high BMI, but the 2AG concentrations in the adipose tissue itself is reduced by 2.3-fold. High circulating levels of 2AG are associated with the accumulation of visceral fat, or fat collection around the organs in the abdomen. This visceral fat is a pro-inflammatory organ on its own and is known to be fed by alcohol use and high fructose corn syrup. Overactivation of CB1R in fat cells induces fat accumulation. Overall, the ECS is being considered as a good pharmacologic target for treating obesity and related diseases, but there are no drugs on the market yet. (At the end of this chapter, you will learn more about toning the ECS without drugs, but using tools at your disposal including food and other integrative strategies.) The American Medical Association has suggested that BMI only be used in conjunction with other valid measures as body shapes and types across ethnic groups/race, gender, age-span and sex should should be included in criteria to determine who is labeled obese as a medical term.

Endocannabinoid Relatives: A Family of Compounds

In addition to ECBs and their protein receptors there are other receptors involved in ECS signaling. These components combined have been called the endocannabinoidome, a network made of other lipid (fat-based) chemicals, enzymes that make and break them and their protein receptors down. Some of these family members work together to help normalize our bodily functions and work in concert with the eCS.

AEA is in the family of ethanolamines, containing compounds with various carbon chain lengths: OEA; PEA, SEA. These are related in that they are all broken down by the same enzyme—FAAH. OEA is known to help ramp-up fat burning through activation of a receptor called PPAR-alpha. Appetite has also been linked to OEA: As OEA levels go up, hunger goes down.[ ] PEA has been shown to have effects on fat metabolism, have anti-inflammatory effects but not shown to have direct effects on appetite.

There is less information about SEA, but this compound and the other ethanolamines do not directly bind the cannabinoid receptors. They are labeled entourage compounds, meaning they may be acting synergistically to affect biochemistry. There is also a family of 2AG-like compounds, the acyl-glycerols, with various chain lengths: 2PG and 2LG are also are considered to have entourage effects regarding 2AG.[31]

This entourage effect was first described as how the ethanolamine and acyl-glycerol compounds are competing for the same enzymes that degrade them. If there is more PEA competing with AEA for FAAH, then the levels of AEA might be elevated. Later, this concept has been applied to plant cannabinoids, as the terpenes are thought to enhance or modulate the effects of THC. This has yet to be proven but is a popular topic in the cannabis culture. There are also other flavor compounds (alcohols, ketones, sulfur compounds) that may be modulating the overall cannabis experience!

When I think of entourage, I think about the television dramedy of that name. In this comedy there is a group of childhood friends that follow their famous movie-star friend around. While THC is popular and famous, the terpenes and other compounds do not follow THC around—they each have their own biologic actions in the body. So far, there is mixed evidence from laboratory studies to support the hypothesis that the terpenes enhance THC binding to CBRs.[32-35] The term synergy has long been used to describe the multiplicity of effects of botanical medicines and is a more appropriate term than entourage to use when describing effects of whole plant cannabis.

Other receptors (proteins) that may be chemically activated by cannabinoids include transient receptor potential (TRP) channels, which are gateways for calcium, sodium, chloride, and potassium to get into cells. TRP is like the electrical charge in nerve and tissue signaling. The activation of TRPV1 by AEA on neurons has been shown to reduce some types of pain. TRPV1 is also found on smooth muscle tissue and the cells that line the blood vessels (endothelial cells). There are also orphan G

protein-coupled, called orphans because their native endogenous ligand*
has not been discovered; GPR55 and GPR18 are being considered as part
of the endocannabinoidome.**

Further complicating the network complexity of ECS signaling is that the
CBRs have been shown to co-join (pharmacology term: heterodimer-
ize) with other receptors in tissues where they both are co-located. This
co-joining affects how proteins send their signals to the internal part of the
cell. The ability to do this enhances the repertoire of what proteins can do,
an example of biology's conservation. It also demonstrates how the ECS is
'playing' with many other systems, what would be expected of a homeostatic paradigm. Some of these protein receptors include melatonin type 1,
dopamine type 2, delta and mu opioid, orexin, somatostatin, GPR55- even
CB2R and CB1R can co-join.[36-38]

Clearly, the control of healthy appetite and metabolism is a constant conversation in the body/mind, with the ECS acting as a primary mediator
across the brain/gut connection. There is additionally the concerted effort
of the rest of the endocannabinoidome, the extending family of proteins,
chemical signalers, and downstream effects that keep us in good working
order. There are important roles for addressing whole person health by optimizing nutrition and our relationship with food, improving stress resilience to aid digestion, modulating anxiety so that we can normalize hunger,
and supporting the microbiome. When treating the GI system, it is integral
to remember that we are complex creatures and a systems approach is most
expedient when health needs arise.

---

* "A ligand is a natural or man-made substance that binds selectively to its receptor on the surface of a cell by bumping on and producing a vibration to open the
doorway to a cell." The receptor transmits this message from the cell surface to
the interior which can in some cases dramatically changes the state of the cell
Candace Pert, Molecules of Emotion: Why You Feel the Way You Feel: Simon and
Schuster. Dec 2016.

** The endocannabinoid "ome" is the ECS as defined previously, plus a spectrum
of other bioactive lipid molecules that make up a network of mediators, their enzymes, and targets.

Mechanical Function of the Gut

I had just returned from a beautiful, long, and gentle hike gaining 1000 ft. in the mountains of northern New Mexico. My heart rate was probably at its max, as I am normally dwelling at sea level, and went up to 8,000 feet. Musing about my energy expenditure (those mitochondria were pumping to make ATP!) to make it up the hill, I noticed that on the way down I started feeling the first pangs of hunger. This feeling is associated with what is called the migrating motor complex (MMC). The MMC is a cyclic contraction starting in the top part of the stomach, the site where gastrin is secreted in the stomach. (Remember this chemical stimulates hunger in the brain.)

This cyclic contraction is a slow wave of electrical stimulation of the smooth muscle in the gut. The electric signal is delivered by the vagus nerve which supplies nerve signals to all of our internal organs. This wanderer, as the vagus nerve is known, is the gut-brain axis communication highway, relaying with the enteric nervous system (ENS). The ENS has more neurons than found in your spine and uses more than 30 neurotransmitters! The contraction starts with the stomach secretions then moves down the GI to the duodenum and small intestines. The role of the MMC is to continually sweep the digestive tract of debris, or leftovers, from the last food we ate; consider it GI housekeeping. Without this normal sweeping function disorders can develop such as: belching, poor digestion, nausea and/or vomiting, gastritis, and bacterial overgrowth (resulting in diarrhea/constipation and/or alternating of the two: the definition of irritable bowel syndrome, IBS).

Our GI's got rhythm! And, you guessed it, CBRs are involved. In general, activation of cannabinoid receptors has been thought to be beneficial for gut pain/discomfort, particularly when related to dysfunction of ENS, our gut's brain. This is where cannabinoid receptors are primarily found but the ECS signals all along the GI tract, regulating motility, acid and fluid release, dilation of blood vessels, nerve conduction, and muscle contraction, along with food intake. Further, the ECS also modulates endocrine cells, cells that secrete chemicals mediating the endocrine and nervous system, specifically those that secrete insulin, which controls blood sugar levels.

Body/Mind Interface #1

Do you ever feel anxious when you feel a hunger pang or out-of-sorts in any other way? I'm going to challenge you. The next time you feel this, try to tune into the feeling. Think of it as described, nerve- stimulated contractions at the top of your stomach (just at the base of your ribcage, just under your heart). Think of the specialized cells that secrete stomach acid and gastrin. Try to relax that part of your body and imagine you are opening a portal from your throat down to that area. As you breathe in, you relax all of the surrounding structures, including all of your abdomen. You feel contraction of the smooth muscle and you should be able to follow it a bit deeper in your belly.

See if you can separate 4 phases of the MMC:

1. No activity or feelings
2. Random contractions
3. A burst of contractions that are longer and stronger
4. Rapid decrease of contractions

By noticing this, you are tuning into the body/mind. You are connecting biological processes with feelings and thoughts. You are gaining interoception or wisdom into your felt state. You are learning your internal perceptions and what they signal to the body. Once your MMC has finished its cycle, it is likely to be repeated every 1.5–2 hours between meals. This is a good reason to leave plenty of time between meals (at least 3–5 hours), so the gut can sweep itself in this way. Food sitting too long in the digestive tract can overfeed the bacteria, ferment, and cause excessive gas or abdominal pain.

Once the cycle is over, what you feel is the homeostasis of the ECS. Close your eyes and embrace the bliss! Overactivity of the MMC or delays in gastric emptying can lead to nausea, pain, and vomiting. Antagonists of the serotonin receptor in the gut, such as ondansetron (Zofran), abolishes the gastric component of phase 3 of the MMC (the stronger burst of contractions). This is a primary means of trying to treat nausea and vomiting.

The GI Has Rhythm

What you feel during digestion are the effects of the neurotransmitter acetylcholine (ACh) which stimulates the smooth muscle tissue and other selected cells in the upper stomach such as parietal cells (ACh is discussed further in Chapters Sleep and Forget). CB1R is found at the terminals of the vagus nerve, touching the stomach muscle and on the acid-secreting parietal cells. On nerve cells, CB1R is gating electrical transmission of signals from other neurochemicals (in this case acetylcholine but also serotonin, dopamine, glutamate, gamma-aminobutyric acid [GABA]). AEA is released on demand by these stomach contractions, then signaling to the vagus nerve that the stomach got the message and to stop sending the signal to contract the muscle or secrete acid. This describes how the ECS is responsible for the negative feedback loop resulting in inhibiting gastric motility.

AEA and CB1R are also involved in gastric emptying.[39] Once we have eaten some food, stomach acid is needed to break apart proteins, so there is a short holding time in the stomach. Next the mixture of food, acid, mucus, or chyme has to continue its journey down the intestines so that we can assimilate and absorb the nutrients. Some people experience delayed gastric emptying. The neurotransmitter serotonin, and also antidepressants that are selective serotonin reuptake inhibitors (SSRIs), can increase the strength and frequency of the MMC below the level of the stomach. Just beneath the stomach in the duodenum, sodium bicarbonate (an acid neutralizer) pancreatic enzymes and bile (from the gall bladder) are being released to further simplify carbohydrates and proteins so we can easily assimilate them for growth and energy.

On parietal cells, the CB1R is associated with effects on secretion of stomach acid.[40] Acid release by parietal cells is a requirement for breaking down of proteins into simpler chains of amino acids. But when there is excessive acid, tissue damage, ulcers, and acid reflux (heartburn) occur. THC can facilitate acetylcholine signaling and thereby facilitate secretions, but at high doses, THC is more likely to be anticholinergic (inhibiting secretions, as what happens with dry mouth often experienced with cannabis, particularly inhaled). This is another example of the biphasic effects of THC. It appears that it can inhibit the breakdown of ACh at low doses, increasing levels of grehlin to stimulates hunger and assisting in maintenance of energy balance or enhancing appetite.

Another important and potent trigger of acid release is the neuro-endocrine chemical called histamine. You have experienced histamine with a runny nose from allergies, or through a reaction to an insect bite. Too much histamine is pro-inflammatory; just the right amount is needed for necessary physiologic functions. Histamine acts on nearby tissues by rapidly dilating blood vessels, constricting airway tubes, and contracting smooth muscle cells. Histamine is related to intestinal cramping and diarrhea. Primarily produced by immune cells, mast cells, and basophils that contain tiny granules of chemicals quickly released to local areas, histamine is also stored in and released on neurons. Histamine is crucial in the immediate response to allergens but can also be involved in chronic inflammation (more on that in Protect).

If the stomach is not emptying or is delayed in emptying, this is a condition called gastroparesis. This slowed emptying can be attributed to high blood sugar, nerve damage that impairs GI motility, and lack of stress resilience. Since the ECS is primarily involved in the feedback loop that slows down motility, there is the potential that cannabis could exacerbate this problem. What is needed in this case is ECS toning and to produce GI movement or a prokinetic agent. There are plenty of these found in nature (discussed at the end of the chapter).

Cyclic vomiting is a disorder with recurrent episodes of severe nausea and vomiting interspersed with symptom free periods. A form of cyclic vomiting called cannabis hyperemesis syndrome (CHS) is plaguing cannabis users, consisting of recurring episodes of nausea, vomiting, abdominal pain, and associated dehydration, sending many cannabis users to the emergency room. Strongly correlated is that victims of CHS report that their pain is relieved by hot showers. It is not known exactly how or why cannabis causes this syndrome for some, but if this is the true diagnosis, it should clear up after discontinuation of cannabis use. According to a 2022 survey and investigation into CHS, about 87% of patients improve after cessation of cannabis.[41]

For those who continue to suffer from CHS symptoms after discontinuing cannabis use, there is likely a different diagnosis. CHS is usually a rapid onset of symptoms, occurring over 1 week with absence of symptoms in between episodes. Many patients report that it is worse in the morning, similar to the morning sickness of early pregnancy. A study of genetics in individuals with CHS revealed that there may be mutations in genes not directly related to the ECS that may put individuals at risk for developing this syndrome including COMT, TRPV1, DRD2, and CYP2C9 metabolizing enzyme. However, these are preliminary findings.[ ]

Case in Point

My patient was a 28-year-old female with a diagnosis of ulcerative colitis two years prior. She had her colon removed, so was wearing a colostomy bag. (Stop for a minute and think about that trauma! Medical trauma can be a huge piece of our stories and we will address it more in depth in Chapters 3 and 5: Relax and Forget.) The first time I saw her, she was not having any severe pain but had been referred to me by the pain specialist I work closely with who wanted her cannabis use evaluated.

She reported that she had used cannabis during her illness and surgeries for pain and anxiety. She said that she mainly used a vape pen (see box 1.4), but also ate cannabis gummies at night. I recommended that she discontinue the use of the vape pen in favor of using a lower-potency vaporized cannabis, and to include an oral cannabis liquid as a means of bringing it directly to her digestive tract, for the potential anti-inflammatory and benefit on visceral sensitivity (pain in the internal organs).

BOX 1.4   VAPE PENS: Concentrated forms of cannabis, like those found in vape pens, are associated with a higher incidence of mental and physical health problems. They may lead to a higher risk of developing acute adverse effects, such as paranoia, psychosis, and cannabis hyperemesis syndrome. While most cannabis flower is around 20-25% THC, concentrates can be up to 90% THC! The perceived low risk of both cannabis and concentrated vape pens as a means of consumption, may bring a false sense of security about health effects. It can seem to be particularly appealing for those looking for a "healthier" way to use cannabis (not smoking). However, vaping of highly concentrated products (such as dabbing or using wax) can be associated with acute lung injury and often involves high-potency forms of cannabis, exposing you to several acute and long-term health risks including downregulation of the ECS. Vaping concentrates is not safe or effective medicine! There are a lot of great vaporizers for cannabis flower (dry vaping). Consider investing in this tool if you are either a cannabis smoker, vape pen other methods to inhale concentrates. Concentrates may be referred to as rosin, dabs' oil, concentrates, and extracts appearing as a thick liquid to a firm, almost glassy solid. They can contain up to 90% THC, compared to 10%-20% in the dry herb. Dry vaping allows for the full enjoyment and benefits of the terpenes, or the essential oil component of cannabis, in its natural state. These compounds are destroyed with combustion (smoking) and can be lost or changed during the process of concentrating cannabis or with high temperatures of vaping. The bioactivity of terpenes is retained with vaporization. Give up the harsh, save your lungs, and protect your ECS!

The reason for discontinuing the vape pen is due to the biphasic effects of THC on pain; vape pens are at a potency beyond the therapeutic window for pain.[42] She returned 2 years later, having been recently hospitalized for a flare of her GI symptoms and abdominal pain was reduced by taking hot showers. I inquired about her vape pen use, and she claimed she was not using it much (I learned later from her family that this was not accurate). She had been treated for small intestinal bacterial overgrowth (SIBO) so I prescribed a restorative protocol for her GI system and reinforced the importance not using the vape pen. I also suggested a CHS diagnosis since she mentioned relief from hot showers, but she was not open to this potential diagnosis. Her anxiety was so high she did not feel like she could withdraw cannabis use.

Six months later, she was experiencing ongoing and worsening pain, a follow-up surgery and using oxycodone to control her pain. She says that cannabis is not helping her pain, that she only uses it for anxiety, and continues to dismiss the idea that she may have CHS. After another 6 months, she returned to tell me that she read about CHS on Reddit and is convinced that this is her diagnosis. She is ready to break the cycle and tapered her cannabis use by 90%. She is still administering it using a vape pen. Her family reports that she had been using the vape once per hour all day. We discuss alternatives for helping with her anxiety, and I provide her a handout on supporting and toning the endocannabinoid system.

This patient ended up going to rehab because the pain management specialists were convinced that she was opioid-seeking. She had increased opioids up to about 150 morphine milligram equivalents per day and had numerous emergency room visits for her pain. Discontinuing cannabis resolved all of her pain, nausea, and vomiting. While all ended well for her eventually, there was a 2-year span where she suffered needlessly from CHS.

Women's Health

Although 50% of both sexes report some disordered GI function, more women than men seek healthcare for GI dysfunction. While there is some speculation that one reason for this is that men seek healthcare less than women in general, the hormone balance (or estradiol in general) can affect this area of women's health. There is an association between being a woman and experiencing irritable bowel syndrome (IBS), irritable bowel disease (IBD), constipation and gall bladder problems. On a monthly basis, hormonal changes and prostaglandin production prior to menstrual flow can trigger bowel contractions resulting in diarrhea. It is also more common for women in perimenopause to start having IBS and gall bladder problems or see these worsen. These conditions can be accompanied by increases in abdominal distension, bloating and gas, constipation, and/or diarrhea and pain. This type of disordered GI function often co-occurs with back pain.

IBS is a functional disorder of the bowel associated with altered bowel movements (either diarrhea (IBS-D) or constipation (IBS-C) or alternating between the two), abdominal pain, and spasms. Patients with IBS-D have shorter cycles of the MMC during the day (but not necessarily at night) and are more likely to have diarrhea-predominant IBS. Regardless of type, this condition is characterized by visceral hypersensitivity, where pain is magnified: what should not be painful is painful. IBS can be triggered by antibiotic use, food poisoning, and is associated with anxiety, depression and H. pylori infection. Patients with any type of IBS have higher levels of motilin, a hormone that is released in the upper part of the small intestine that stimulates small intestine motility (phase 3 of the MMC). Therapies to treat IBS by gastroenterologists include antidiarrheal drugs, antispasmodic drugs, fiber, antidepressants, antibiotic therapy for SIBO, opioids (to slow gut motility), and anticholinergic drugs—but often with low-level results and common recurrence.

There is also the potential that too much motility, as in IBS-D, can be related to inflammation in the gut, whereby CB2R signaling is implicated. Targeting the ECS directly with THC can sometimes be helpful for slowing motility as well as addressing inflammation and imbalances in our bacteria communities or microbiome. There needs to be a deep dive into underlying causes for anyone suffering from IBS, as it is multifaceted and complex. Functional testing for bacterial overgrowth, presence of H. pylori infection, pancreatic insufficiency, dietary influences, underlying past trauma, and acute stress can all be significant players that need to be addressed with GI dysfunction such as IBS. There is not usually one quick fix.

Slowing GI motility with THC can be helpful for some patients with diarrhea, as THC both slows peristalsis and provides some pain benefit or symptom relief. For constipation, targeting the TRPV1 receptor is strategy, and the best compound for this is capsaicin from hot peppers. (Cannabidiol also binds the TRPV1 receptor and has been reported to cause loose stools at high dose.) Capsaicin can be used in enteric-coated capsules to desensitize this receptor, which can decrease visceral pain and some other symptoms (e.g., bloating).[43, 44] Topical application of capsaicin has been shown to benefit CHS and also can help ease cramping in IBS. Addressing the microbiome is also important.

Speaking of bowel movements, when is the last time you looked at your poop? You can score it using the Bristol stool chart to describe them.* The shape, type, and density can tell a lot about what is happening in your GI tract. The ideal poop is type 3 or 4. See if you can notice whether making changes to your diet can change your poop type! More fiber helps the GI move better, and simply drinking more and exercising can help with constipation.

Irritable bowel disease (IBD) consists of an inflammatory underlying disorder and includes the diagnoses of Crohn's disease (CD) and ulcerative colitis (UC). Many patients with IBD report improvement in symptoms with cannabis use, including improvements in pain, reduced number of bowel movements per day, and improved appetite. However, in one study of 389 individuals with IBD, who did or did not use cannabis, cannabis users reported more abdominal pain, joint pain, gas, and feeling of the need to pass stool, even when none was present.[45] Given the inflammatory component of IBD, cannabinoid medicine may be an appropriate add-on for this patient population, particularly if lacking good symptom control using conventional medical approaches. However, the clinical evidence is not there to support cannabis as a singular approach to treating this disorder but it may help address general well-being and quality of life. Remember that the anti-inflammatory effects of CB2R function in the GI is an important therapeutic target (THC activates this receptor, CBD does not. See Chapter: Protect). Dietary cannabinoids can be a good approach for toning the ECS in this disorder. It is important to note that THC has a biphasic effect on pain (see Chapter 5: Forget). Targeting the ECS for IBD needs proven approaches and more research. Cannabis may help some patients by reducing symptom severity.

---

* You can access a visual and description of the types here: *https://www.webmd. com/digestive-disorders/poop-chart-bristol-stool-scale*

THC binds to and activates both CB1R and CB2R, handy for impacting both the nervous (in this case the ENS) and immune system contributions. There is a mistaken idea that CBD is an agonist or activates the CB2R, but this was **herban legend #1** described in the introduction (page 4).[46] CBD has been shown to bind both CB1R and CB2R, but not as an agonist or an activator of ECS function. It may bind to CBR, but it more likely inactivates CB1R and has little potency at CB2R. Rather, CBD may impair the ability of endocannabinoids or THC to activate the receptors (known as an inverse agonist or negative allosteric modulator). One example of this is the ability of CBD to block migration of cells in cultured cell experiments. CB1R is known to be involved in the chemotaxis of immune cells, but in culture, CBD blocks this effect.[47] CBD has been shown to have anti-inflammatory potential in animal models and in cell cultures, but there is no evidence of this, yet, in humans. If there is a dose of CBD that may be anti-inflammatory, it is unknown. Doses of 150 mg of CBD are being tried in a couple of clinical trials as an anti-inflammatory and for sparing of steroid use.

While on the topic of CBD, since it is not engaging the ECS directly, CBD is not an analgesic, or a pain reliever like THC. The primary disorder that CBD has been proven to work for is intractable childhood epilepsies. There is an FDA-approved drug for this indication (Epidiolex™). There have been a few small studies of CBD for pain, but none of them showed significant benefit, including a meta-analysis and systematic review of the available research.[48, 49] There is insufficient evidence, including my own personal clinical observations after working with chronic pain patients for the past 12 years, that CBD treats pain. Cannabigerol (CBG), another minor cannabinoid is currently under investigation for the ability to stimulate appetite.

Disorders of Eating

Anorexia nervosa (AN) is a nutritional disorder where due to a lack of fuel, the body burns its own muscle tissue (after all the fat is gone) to try to maintain body weight—but there is a severe loss of fat and muscle mass. There have only been a few organized studies for testing whether cannabis can be helpful in this disorder. The ECS is implicated in AN, as blood levels of AEA in women with AN are significantly higher than that of healthy controls.[50] High anandamide levels also correlate with low levels of leptin. Dronabinol (synthetic THC, marketed as Marinol) was shown to help with weight gain, but higher doses of THC were not helpful (an example of biphasic effects). There is a need for more research into targeting the ECS for this disorder, but persons suffering from AN need a trauma-informed care approach along with multiple integrative approaches to recovery (more on this in Chapters 3 and 5: Relax and Forget). Cannabis is not a panacea but may help stimulate appetite and aid with weight gain. A recent study has suggested that psilocybin, a serotonin receptor agonist from Psilocybe mushrooms may be effective for AN.[51]

Binge-eating disorder is an inability to stop eating even when full, occurring at least once a week for three months. This is the most common eating disorder in women, and can be deadly if not treated. It can be a component of AN-related bingeing/purging. Cannabis could be helpful for stress management in this diagnosis, but there is also the potential for exacerbating the problem by promoting appetite.

Binge eating is another situation (such as with obesity) where blockade of the CB1R might be helpful, but until drugs are developed that will *not* cross over into the brain, the depression risk is too great. A minor cannabinoid known as THCV (a different carbon chain length analog of THC) is an alternative, minor cannabinoid with evidence that it acts as an antagonist at CB1R. I don't recommend trying this on your own. Personal experience and my substantial experience working with patients suggests that THCV may also have negative effects on mood, causing *dysphoria* rather than the *euphoria* commonly associated with THC and effects on balance. THCV was found to be helpful in mice to reduce body fat content, and decrease leptin in obese animals.[52]

Chemotherapy-induced nausea and vomiting (CINV) is a common experience for cancer patients receiving IV or oral chemotherapy treatments. CINV is the most common side effect in chemotherapy-treated patients, associated with loss of appetite, weight loss, and loss of quality of life.[53] Most conventional CINV treatment is use of serotonin receptor (in the gut) antagonist drugs. Improving appetite is a starring role for cannabis and can be a valuable herbal ally for chemotherapy-treated cancer patients. Synthetic THC (dronabinol/Marinol) was trialed for CINV, given at a dose of 2.5 mg twice per day, either alone or in combination with megestrol acetate (an analog of the hormone progesterone). In this study, THC was not found to be effective for CINV.[54]

Cannabis is known as one of the oldest remedies for nausea and vomiting.[55] Patients with cancer who access and use locally sourced cannabis overwhelmingly report favorable results. It could be that the whole plant, other doses than those in the clinical trial, or administering cannabis by inhalation may be better options for this patient group. Given the overall potential benefits for patients with cancer for quality of life, cannabis is worth a try, and with proper medical guidance can be used effectively to help prevent cachexia (loss of skeletal muscle mass that is not fully reversed by conventional nutritional support), which has been associated with poorer survival.[ ] Low dose of THC may help with appetite without causing sedation. Everyone can have different experiences with ingesting THC in a cannabis edible or liquid, due to liver enzymes and how THC is metabolized in the liver. The liver makes a metabolite of THC, 11-hydroxy THC that is known to be potentially more potent than THC itself. If you have an enzyme system that makes a lot of this metabolite or makes it rapidly, it can potentially lead to a more intense effect that desired. This is one rationale for starting with a very low dose of THC.

The Other "Us": Microbiome

This chapter is not complete without returning to think about the vast majority of who we are: our microbiome. They, the hundreds of species of bacteria, fungi, protozoa, viruses, and things unnamed inside our GI tract, outnumber our own cells by ten-to-one. They are all intimately involved in human health and homeostasis. First, they have trained our immune system. They are all over us, literally, everywhere our inside world meets the outside world (thanks to one of my teachers, Becky Love, for that imagery). They live on our outer surfaces, too. They form a community in which we live as symbiotes—a mutually beneficial relationship. One gift we receive is help with keeping things that are non-self out, to avoid infection or self-attack. A unique crosstalk exists between our microbiome and our immune system to facilitate this symbiosis. (See Chapter 4: Protect.)

It's the early window of exposure to microbes, soon after birth and in our infancy, that determines our future health. Imbalances in the microbiome, known as dysbiosis, has been associated with broad health outcomes such GI and mood disorders. Early life is the time that our immune system is in training; it is being programmed by our environment. Our GI tube is rich with ECS function, in the nerves, intestinal epithelial cells, secretory cells, smooth muscle responsible for peristalsis, and in the huge immune tissue lining our entire digestive tract. (How interesting that so much of our immune tissue is so close to the outside world!) One of the access points for the outside world to the inside world, or transducers of the outside world to the inside world, is the microbiome lining the gut.

Just underneath the microbiota and a mucus layer are the intestinal epithelial cells. There are tight connections between these epithelial cells in the gut so that foreign proteins can't get in. The CB2R is here to be in more direct connection with the outside world. The CB2R is found predominantly in the large immune system that lines the gut. AEA, 2AG, and PEA (palmitoyl-ethanolamine) are all produced in the gut, helping gut permeability (helping to heal the tight connections of epithelial cells) and signaling in the entero-endocrine cells. These cells are hybrid neuron/secretory cells. They respond to, and in some cases secrete, neurotransmitters such as serotonin, gastrin, and other key hormone modulators, and ECS signaling, providing the bridge for the gut-brain axis. (More on this in Chapter Relax.)

Just below the epithelial cells, in the mucosa, the largest collection of our immune system, Peyer's patches line the small intestine, nodules of immune cells—at-the-ready. These patches are the immune sensors of the GI tract, numbering about 100 when we are at peak performance (numbers decline with age).

B cells are important players on the immune team as they secrete IgA antibodies, up to several grams per day. This IgA, in turn, helps to keep our microbiome balanced with appropriate diversity. In other words, it takes all kinds! The more diversity of fiber that we have in our diet, the more diverse our microbiome. These critters need food too—what we eat fuels our bugs and our cells.

Some things that can go wrong are death to a lot of bacteria (with overuse of antibiotics), imbalances in bacteria, inflammation leading to leaky gut—all associated with inflammation. ECS can come to the rescue as the CB2R is intended to turn down the noise on inflammation. By activating the CB2R we can help to accomplish this, but it takes a more comprehensive approach to a healthy microbiome (see below) by addressing underlying causes and also taking a deep dive into your health history, your nutrition, lifestyle habits and stress management. The ultimate goal is to get your cells into homeostasis.

We need things from our microbiome, such as short chain fatty acids (SCFAs: butyrate, acetate, propionate) neurotransmitters (serotonin, GABA, dopamine), vitamins (B12, thiamine, folate, vitamin K), and immune surveillance. We need to feed them by minimizing carbohydrates, avoiding artificial sweeteners and eating plenty and diverse fiber (20–30 grams per day—make an exercise of counting how much fiber you get per day). Because microbiome disturbances can promote immune dysregulation and lead to disease (such as IBD), functional testing of the microbiome can be useful. Treating overgrowth of certain bacteria or yeast helps you keep inflammation at bay and promotes balance in the gut microbiome.

Specifically for the ECS, *Lactobacillus acidophilus* has been shown to upregulate the CB2R and opioid receptors on gut epithelium, an intervention for visceral pain, as well modulating immune tissue function in the gut.[56] *Akkermansia muciniphila* (an anti-inflammatory species in the gut that normally lives there) upregulates ECBs, while dysbiosis (microbiome imbalances) depletes the levels of ECBs. This disruption of the balance of the microbiome is linked to disease and neuroinflammation. ECBs are necessary for the immune homeostasis in the GI tract as well as for peristalsis.[57]

Maintenance of homeostasis in the gut is fundamental to health, and the ECS's role is a gatekeeper for maintaining the tight junctions, minimizing inflammation and bringing dysbiosis to equilibrium after antibiotic use.[58]

Imbalances in the gut microbiome can arise from antibiotic use, probiotic use, high "bad" fat (as in saturated and omega-6 fatty acids), and high-sugar diets. When things are out of control, the microbiome can adhere to the epithelial layer, forming a biofilm that is resistant to being killed off by bacteria. These manipulations also can change our ECS, such as affecting the expression of the CB1R or CB2R. Toning the ECS is a key to help keep our gut in homeostasis. If you undergo any therapy to treat SIBO, find an integrative practitioner who can help you rebuild your microbiome and gut health. There are four important process steps: 1) normalizing motility, 2) dietary interventions, 3) breaking down biofilms using natural biocides, and 4) rebuilding the microbiome.

The microbiome is implicated in gastrointestinal cancer, obesity and diabetes, gut permeability, IBS, IBD, hyperlipidemia, atherosclerosis, liver disease, mental health, and stress resilience.[59] Attention to this part of who we are is essential for a balanced ECS in our GI system, as well as whole person health and longevity.

Naturopathic/Integrative/Functional Approaches
Care of the ECS

Dietary cannabinoids are found in non-cannabis botanicals and can help to tone our ECS, particularly in the gut. Supportive foods include polyunsaturated fats, particularly omega-3 fatty acids (FAs) that also have cardiovascular and neurological health benefits. The ideal ratio of omega 3:6 fatty acids is 1:1 while a typical American diet is 1:10. In addition, too little omega-3 FAs lead to impaired glucose in skeletal muscle (leading to putting on more fat), stimulating osteoclast proliferation (which breaks down bone), and generating pro-inflammatory compounds. Hemp seeds, flax seed, chia seeds, and walnuts all contain ECS-enhancing FAs. Olive oil also contains ethanolamine, a compound needed to make AEA. Omega-3 sources include salmon, mackerel, herring, oysters, sardines, flax seed, walnuts, and chia seed. (More in Chapter Forget.)

Terpenes

Limonene has been used for treating acid reflux. Betacaryophyllene is toning for the immune system in the gut.

Measuring Allostatic Load

Metabolic assessments for AL associated with "Eat" include: serum lipids (best when blood is drawn after fasting overnight) including high-density lipoprotein (HDL—considered good cholesterol, unless it is too high), low-density lipoprotein (LDL—genetics of these proteins can indicate our risk for cardiovascular diseases) and triglycerides; insulin resistance (IR—insulin can be measured too), BMI, and waist-to-hip ratio (WHR) and glucose/hemoglobin A1C (glucose load over time). Increased AL can be measured in lab tests by increases in all of these markers excepting HDL, where too low of a value is not beneficial. There are various specialty tests for measuring elements of the microbiome, dysbiosis (breath and stool tests), inflammation, and permeability in the gut.

Herbal Allies

Prokinetic herbs: Useful for bloating, burping, acid reflux, nausea, and abdominal pain. If your body is unable to move food, waste, and bacteria down and out, you're likely to end up with a problem with the ileocecal valve. A bacteria and parasite coinfection will develop and result in bacterial overgrowth. Keep in mind that your MMC is critical in this development. Anytime we slow down the MMC or it becomes dysregulated, you are essentially slowing down that sweeping cleansing action, which is an integral part of gastrointestinal health and also immune system health.

Zingiber officinale: Ginger accelerates gastric emptying and promotes the MMC. Magnolia bark (magnolol and honokiol have been shown in animal studies to speed up intestinal transit), turkey rhubarb, bitter orange peel (immature) also promote the MMC.

Triphala: An herbal combination of three fruits used in Ayurvedic medicine: amalaki, bibhitaki, and haritaki. It is considered a gentle bowel tonic, intended to support digestion and gut health.

Curcuma longa: Turmeric is found in the spice known as curry. It is a yellow pigment and can be useful for reducing intestinal inflammation and IBS symptoms; it contains the active ingredient curcumin, which has been shown to inhibit the COX2 enzyme (same action as ibuprofen).[60]

Cinnamomum: Cinnamon is the bark from a tree found in Indonesia; it is a strong spice that has been named as one of the highest antioxidant capacities of any plant. It has a long history of use as a digestive aid. It may also help lower glucose levels and reduce inflammation in the body. It can also help make the GI "friendly" for the good bacteria or adaptogenic for the microbiome.

Myristica fragrans: Nutmeg is another spice, from the seed of a tree found in Malaysia. It is often used along with cinnamon in pumpkin pie and eggnog. It has been used traditionally to help ease indigestion and diarrhea, but at high doses can be toxic. A compound in nutmeg has been shown to inhibit the enzymes that degrade ECBs.

Mentha piperita (**peppermint**) and *Carum carvi* (**Indian cumin, caraway seed or oil**) slow the MMC by causing smooth muscle relaxation.

Avoid protein pump inhibitors (PPIs): A PPI is a drug that treats heartburn or high stomach acidity. Used in the long term (>6 weeks), PPIs can impair nutrient bioavailability such as magnesium and calcium and B12 This, in turn, can lead to kidney problems, osteoporosis, B12 deficiency, and more. There is also evidence that PPIs may contribute to cognitive decline and so should be used for no longer than 6 weeks while treating the underlying cause of the GI issue. If you are on a PPI and want to discontinue you will likely need to taper off and work with a qualified provider to address any ongoing hyperacidity of the stomach.

Treat the microbial community: There is evidence that IBS is connected to SIBO more than 60% of the time, and that SIBO can be associated with a prior food poisoning event. *Escherichia coli* (or *E. coli*) and *Klebsiella* infection are two bacteria that are associated with the release of an endo-toxin that our immune system reacts to. Our immune system can also attack itself in a process called molecular mimicry (autoimmunity) our immune system also starts to produce an antibody to something that is self. This causes problems for the gut lining, leading to leaky gut, and problems with the ENS in the gut leading to impaired peristalsis. Diagnosis of SIBO is imperative and a qualified practitioner will use breath testing for hydrogen, hydrogen sulfide, and methane gas. This result guides the specific treatment. Notably, after treating SIBO, rebuilding the gut is important. If there is an autoimmune element to the IBS, this also needs to be addressed. Finding a trusted healthcare provider who is well-versed in this type of integrative, naturopathic, and functional approach to treatment is important!

Supplements

Antihistamine herbs: *Urticia diocia* is stinging nettle. This common herb in natural medicine may also be a natural antihistamine and help to calm mast cells that line the gut.[61] These cells are prime for producing histamine, which can exacerbate or even cause digestive problems.

Quercetin: This is an antioxidant found naturally in onions, apples, and other produce. Another known mast cell inhibitor, quercetin stabilizes the cell membrane of the mast cell the mast cell then does not spill histamine as easily.[62]

Bromelain: Bromelain is a mixture of enzymes commonly found in pineapples, but you can also take it as a supplement. This can be helpful in SIBO and also as a digestive aid.

Probiotics: The best way to boost the microbiome is to ingest prebiotic foods. Eating a wide variety of fruits, vegetables, and grains, along with specific types of fiber, helps normalize the microbiota in many cases. There is a lot of testing available to learn what microbes, and in what abundance, are in the gut, but the interpretation of results lags behind the development of tests. In the future we will likely be able to target specific imbalances by providing specific organisms (taking probiotics). Some good fiber sources include beans, onions, asparagus, banana, berries, quinoa, and oatmeal.

The bacterial strains *Lactobacillus* and *Bifidobacterium* both produce a calming neurotransmitter, GABA.

Food/Nutrition

Fiber is the best way to treat your GI! Black pepper, oregano, cinnamon, and cloves contain beta-caryophyllene, a CB2R agonist, helping tone this receptor in the gut as a sentinel for inflammation. Sometimes an elimination diet can be helpful to learn about any personal food triggers. We can have food 'sensitivities' that are not like a full blown allergic reaction. Notice if any foods cause you to have runny nose, turn red, increase your heart rate or sneeze.

Yoga/Chakra

The solar plexus, the third or Manipura chakra, is associated with digestion and self-honor. The color associated with this chakra is yellow, as the corresponding element is fire. It is located where a group of our nerves, the celiac plexus exists in the middle of our gut. This chakra is associated with disempowerment and victimization.

Yoga postures for this chakra include any position that works to strengthen the core or the abdominal muscles: paripurna navasana or boat pose, surya namaskar or sun salutation (a pose sequence) and warrior poses are good starting postures. The pranayama kapalabhati or "breath of fire" and other breathing exercises of yoga can help to strengthen the diaphragm and thus digestion. The sacred sound of the universe, chanted as Om, when done to its fullest, will help to tone the vagus nerve, as can the ujjayi breathing technique.

Monitoring Cannabis Effects on Appetite

Trials	Date/ Time	Oral/ Inhaled	Dose/ Product	Last Food (Time)	Desire to Eat (1-10)	1 Hour	2 Hours	3 Hours
1								
2								
3								
4								

Monitoring Cannabis Effects on GI Symptoms

Trials	Date/ Time	Oral/ Inhaled	Dose/ Product	Pain	# of Poops	Quality of Poop	Bloating	Gas
1								
2								
3								
4								

CHAPTER 2:

Sleep

Gartan Mother's Lullaby

Sleep my child, for the red bee hums, the silent twilight falls,
Aoibheall from the grey rock comes, to wrap the world in thrall.
A leanbhan oh, my child, my joy, my love and heart's desire,
The crickets sing you lullaby, beside the dying fire.
Dusk is drawn and the Green Man's thorn is wreathed in rings of fog,
Siabhra sails his boat till morn, along the Starry Bog.
A leanbhan oh, the palely moon hath wreathed her cusp in dew,
And weeps to hear the sad sleep-tune, I sing, my love, to you.
Faintly sweet doth the chapel bell, ring o'er the valley dim,
Tearmann's peasant voices swell, in fragrant evening hymn.
A leanbhan oh, the low bell rings, my little lamb to rest,
And angel-dreams till morning sings, its music in your head.
Sleep oh babe, for the red bee hums the silent twilight's fall,
Aoibheall from the grey rock comes, to wrap the world in thrall.
A leanbhan oh, my child, my joy, my love, my heart's desire,
The crickets sing you lullaby, beside the dying fire.
The crickets sing you lullaby, beside the dying fire.

Herbert Hughes and Seosamh Mac Cathmhaoil, first published in *Songs of Uladh [Ulster]* in 1904 (public domain)

Overview

The sound of a gentle rain. Whispers of crickets. Being rocked (rhythm). Wrapped in arms. Softness, quiet, and dark become our abode. At least in my wildest dreams (pun intended) this is some ideal of how falling asleep should be! Waking refreshed, free of pain, and anticipating another day on the planet is our natural state of health, while insomnia, or the inability to maintain sleep across the night, is the most common sleep disorder that humans are plagued by.

Humans are circadian beings, illustrated by the fact that our bodies have an internal clock. This clock puts us on an approximate 24-hour cycle; we are awake when it is light and asleep when it is dark. This is known as a zeitgeber (German for time-giver), an external or environmental cue that helps to set and regulate our biological rhythms. Exercise, eating, melatonin, cortisol, and dopamine are more zeitgebers. This synchronization of our bodies with the revolving of the earth is survival-based. Circadian (about a day) function in cells, when cultured and treated in a laboratory setting, have also been shown to have rhythm. This is because of clock genes found at the heart of every one of our cells. This kind of timekeeping is found in all higher forms of life and is an integral feature of our biochemistry.

Circadian disruption, which can be caused by even a few days of sleep deprivation, is associated with mood disorder, increases in obesity, high blood pressure, inflammation, and effects on brain regions associated with memory. Disruptions to the 24-hour rhythm alters our allostasis and adds to the wear and tear on our bodies and our brains.

What Is Sleep?

Sleep is an altered state of consciousness where we are not exactly dormant, but most bodily systems are significantly slowed. We have no external activity or conscious interaction with the outside world. We are suspended, yet many physiologic and biochemical functions continue, unbeknownst to us.

Each tissue has its own internal biological clock and there is also a master clock overseeing each of these other timekeepers. Can you guess what organ is an outside regulator of the master clock? (Hint: It is a part of the brain).

It is actually two brain extensions: our eyes and photoreceptors (nerve cells triggered by light) in the retina working as sensory cells. The detection of

Time for a Body Connection Check-in:

First place yourself on the line.

←————————————————————————————————→

++Body Awareness   **Body Detachment++**

For each statement below, assess yourself on this scale:
not at all, a little bit, sometimes, most of the time, all of the
time.

_____ 1. It is difficult for me to identify my emotions.
_____ 2. It is hard for me to express certain emotions.
_____ 3. When I am tense, I take note of where the
        tension is located in my body.
_____ 4. I notice my breathing becoming shallow when I
        am nervous.

For each time you answered not at all, score a zero; a little bit
= 1; some of the time = 2; most of the time = 3; and all of the
time = 4. These questions are part of a larger survey on the
Scale of Body Connection. How do you score? Statements 1
and 2 represent body disconnection (higher score better),
while statements 3 and 4 represent body awareness (lower
score better). Do you think you are improving in
your body awareness? Awareness of the relationships between diet, digestion, and poops can be a
great start!

light or darkness by the retina signals to deeper parts of the brain to turn
on/off clock genes. These genes are what allow for our repair, rest, and re-
cuperation; timekeeping is fundamental to life.

The first relay station for the oncoming dark/light is an area called the suprachiasmatic nuclei (SCN), a collection of about 10,000 nerve cell bodies,
located about 3 centimeters behind the eyes, and behind this is the pineal
organ, or gland, that secretes melatonin. The pineal gland is tightly controlled by the SCN and is a vital part of our internal endocrine calendar.

The ECS machinery for making AEA, PEA, and 2-AG have been detected in the pineal gland of rats![63] We have a plethora of sleep-inducing compounds made by our body. How many ways can this this circadian process and getting sleep go awry and what happens when it does? Sleep disorders are harmful to health because of risks associated with immune function (susceptibility to infection), metabolic syndrome, cancer, and Alzheimer disease (per the American Medical Association).[64]

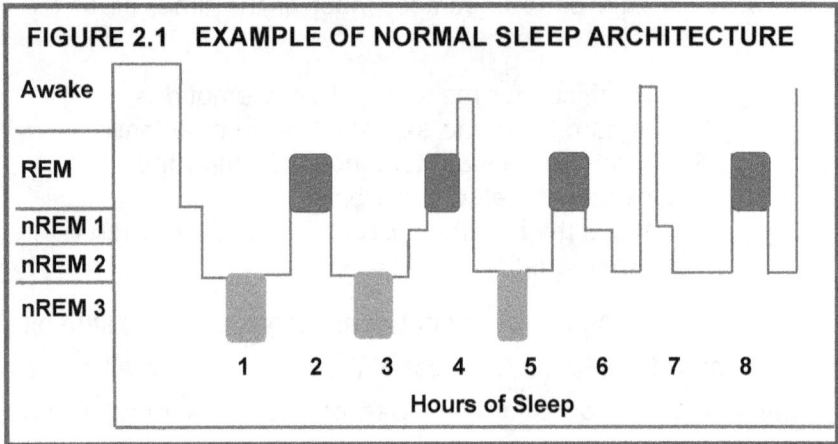

FIGURE 2.1   EXAMPLE OF NORMAL SLEEP ARCHITECTURE

Light comes into the eyes in the morning, activates photoreceptors on the retina which in turn activates the SCN and inhibits the secretion of melatonin. Darkness does the opposite. This describes the basic homeostatic sleep response, necessary for us to survive. We need adequate sleep time for our cognitive, emotional, nervous, immune, cardiovascular—pretty much all of our systems' functioning. We also need a proper quality of sleep for maintaining health and integrating what we learn each day. If we can't get to sleep or stay asleep, we may use sedatives and wake up feeling more like we have been under anesthesia.

There are 4 distinct phases of sleep that define our sleep architecture, and our brain electrical activity modulates them (Figure 2.1). Stage 1 is when you first lie down and start settling in, when you may find your thoughts drifting and slowing; you are dozing off. This should take no more than 15 minutes. Rapid eye movement (REM) occurs between waking and the second stage of sleep, non-REM 1 (NREM1), where our brains produce theta waves, which are slower than the beta/gamma waves of wakefulness or REM sleep. On electrical measurement of brain activity (via electroencephalogram, or EEG), spindles, or brief bursts of electrical energy, thought to be associated with the solidification (or consolidation) of memories of our day are visible.

NREM stages 2 and 3 are the deepest levels of sleep, where we get our most restorative sleep and the brain produces delta waves, or slow-wave sleep. This is also when electrical waves from across all brain areas come together in a slow rhythm. This slow rhythm has been shown to be connected to a pumping action of the watery liquid that circulates around the brain tissue, the cerebrospinal fluid (CSF). This action is associated with the lymphatic system in the brain called glymphatics, discovered in 2012.[65] This helps our brain regions communicate better when we are awake. (The glymphatic system/brain pump will be discussed more in Chapter Forget, where we discuss brain inflammation, cognitive function and the need for this cleaning of brain tissue for homeostasis.) The brain pump and lymph cycle at night is just one reason that this part of the sleep architecture is called restorative.

Deep sleep, the sleep phase which has no REM, is when muscles repair, immune function is strengthened, and tissues regrow. It is also the stage where sleep disorders such as sleepwalking, night terrors, and bedwetting can occur. After NREM2/3, we slowly escalate back out of deep sleep and into REM. REM (25% of sleep time) is also considered restful sleep, but is associated with brain activity or dreaming. Did you know that during REM sleep you are paralyzed? Dreaming aids our ability to organize events in time, or to remember all of the parts we need to know when learning something new (part of the consolidation of memory). It is also responsible for helping us to forget the things that are not essential for us to know. If we remembered everything we saw/heard/experienced every waking moment, we would be driven crazy! This has been suggested to be a critical function of the ECS. Dreaming is also important for our creativity. It has been speculated that the ECS is involved in dreaming.[66] Each night should consist of 4–5 of these complete sleep cycles.

Body/Mind Interface #2: Evaluate Your Relationship with Sleep

1. How do you respond to feeling sleepy?
2. How long does it take you to fall asleep?
3. Do you wake during the night, and if so, how many times? What wakes you?
4. If you wake, do you have a problem getting back to sleep?
5. How many total hours of sleep do you get?
6. Do you wake feeling rested?
7. Do you snore, act out dreams, or have restless leg syndrome?
8. Do you remember dreams?
9. Are you getting sleep prior to midnight?
10. Do you use any type of sleep aids (prescription or over-the-counter?)

- If it takes you more than 30 minutes to fall asleep, if you have difficulty getting back to sleep after waking, or if you are waking excessively, you will likely not wake feeling rested. Your body is not able to repair, and this will promote general inflammation and fatigue in the body.
- If you are not getting a minimum of 7–8 hours of sleep per night, you are unlikely to wake feeling rested and your body may not be completely repairing.
- If you don't go to sleep until after midnight, you may be missing out on the best restorative and healing sleep available.
- If you are using antihistamines or benzodiazepines to help you sleep, you may be harming your brain's health by impairing sleep and depleting acetylcholine.
- If you experience sleep deprivation, this promotes an increase in desire to consume foods for the purposes of pleasure, in the absence of physical hunger (known as hedonic eating as opposed to physiologic hunger or the need for caloric energy).
- Insufficient sleep is a risk factor for obesity, cardiovascular disease, poorer cognitive function, and cognitive decline in later age.
- If you have an undiagnosed or unaddressed sleep disruptor, it is time to address it!

By the end of this chapter, you will have more insight into how your sleep patterns are affecting your health, and some ideas on restoring sleep homeostasis.

Body/Mind Interface 2a

The ability to sleep well can be complicated and sometimes relates to sleep experiences from childhood. Do you remember having sleep problems as a child? One of the things that can enhance our relationship with sleep is the ability to ritualize it as maybe your family did when you were young. For some this may include using cannabis or winding down in another way such as a hot bath, reading etc. . .

In thinking back on your sleep history, was going to bed ever traumatic? Maybe you experienced a fear of the dark, bad dreams, or worry/ruminating about events that held you back from sleeping? Maybe there was food or financial insecurity in your home, and you heard your parents discuss these issues? Bringing this type of experience to our adult consciousness can sometimes help us understand our relationships with sleep in present time and help lead us to solutions by uncovering a piece of the underlying cause.

In a safe and quiet place, close your eyes and allow yourself to drift back to the time of childhood and imagine your sleeping situation. What is the environment where you slept? What noises or smells do you recall? Did you have any type of bedtime ritual such as bathing, being told a story, or getting tucked in by a familiar presence? Did your sleep have an absence of these ritualistic experiences? Did you have trauma around sleep or experience night terrors? Introducing events like these to our current consciousness allows to bring them into the light, first by acknowledging them and then by providing the ability to address them.

Case in Point

My patient is a woman in her forties who was recently diagnosed with early-stage, low-grade breast cancer. Her stated goals for our visit were to "make lifestyle changes to support a stronger immune system, less stress, less inflammation and related disease, improve quality of life, and longevity." She says that she has no health problems (outside of the cancer diagnosis). She has had hip replacements on both sides due to osteoarthritis (no health problems). As I go through the systems review of "eat, sleep, relax, protect, forget" with her, I learn that she thinks she has never had any sleep problems. She reports that she only "needs" about 5 hours of sleep, sleeps from midnight to 5–6 a.m., and does not remember ever sleeping 8 hours at night. She says she thinks she is "wired for stress". The relationship between her sleep quantity/quality, inflammation, stress, arthritis, and cancer is a waving red flag.

I inquired further about how she slept as a child. Her energy and facial expression changes as she starts to recall the impact of growing up with a disabled sister. Her sister was older, and was 100% physically incapacitated from birth. She tells me that she was diagnosed with "nervous stomach" at age 5, and remembers having nausea. Further, she shared that as a young child, she was so fearful about her sister's well-being, that she slept on a couch outside of her sister's room. This was because in her young mind she rationalized that "in case there was a fire," she would be there to save her. For her, there was no conscious awareness around her "stress-wired-ness," her sleep habits and her current diagnosis. The role of trauma in the promotion of inflammation, along with the poor sleep quantity/quality across her life were underlying causes that needed to be addressed to support her healing and to help her reach her stated goals of supporting immunity, decreasing inflammation, and reducing stress. These are all important pieces to address along with any cancer therapy.

The ECS Provides That We Sleep

Our endocannabinoid production has rhythm and has been shown to modulate circadian function in all mammals. The signaling of the ECS that affects our circadian function is in specific parts of the brain. All of the parts of the ECS have been shown to have changes across the day, supporting a link between other circadian regulators, including at our intrinsic clock, the SCN. AEA is considered to be a soporific or sleep-inducer (like chamomile tea in the Beatrix Potter tale of Peter Rabbit). AEA binding to the

CB1R been shown to enhance levels of adenosine* (in a sleep study in rats) and this is one way that it may help to induce sleep. This effect is inhibited by blocking the CB1R, so AEA binding to CB1R enhances adenosine levels, thereby driving sleep. CB1R density in the hippocampus is higher during rodent's inactive phase (during the day for a nocturnal creature) again showing the ECS association with diurnal rhythms.

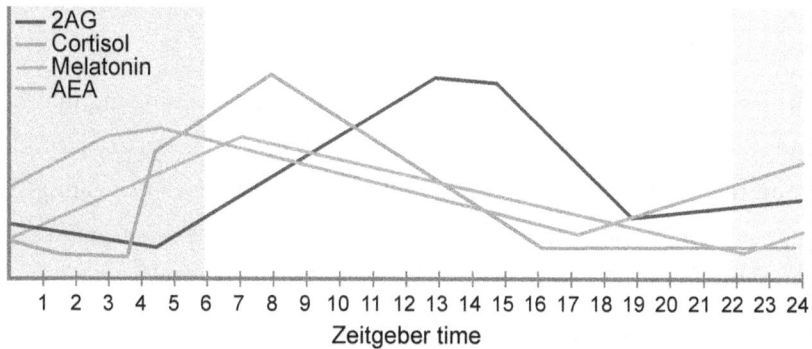

FIGURE 2.2 EXAMPLE OF SLEEP-RELATED HORMONES DAILY FLUCTUATIONS

— 2AG
— Cortisol
— Melatonin
— AEA

1 2 3 4 5 6 7 8 9 10 11 12 13 14 15 16 17 18 19 20 21 22 23 24
Zeitgeber time

AEA production has a normal daily pattern of rising and falling or its own circadian rhythm. Sleep deprivation affects this normal rhythm of AEA production, in which case it may continue to rise across the day, rather than fall in the afternoon. AEA is also likely a modulator of REM sleep as REM phase is associated with levels of AEA going up. 2AG on the other hand is thought to be associated with, or to promote wakefulness, consistent with the fact that it is at its highest levels midday and at its lowest level around 2 a.m. around the time when melatonin is peaking. These endocannabinoid compounds have diurnal rhythms, as do melatonin and cortisol. Figure 2.2 suggests how they vary over the course of a day.

The data on AEA is very small, coming from only 5 subjects at 3 time points.[67] Note that when sleep-deprived, 2AG levels will be higher than with adequate sleep, helping to explain the hedonic eating that has been associated with sleep deprivation.[68] Timing of sleep, as well as the number

---

* You have experienced antagonizing adenosine if you are a coffee drinker or use other caffeine! This blocking action prevents drowsiness.

of hours of sleep, affect the ECS. Notice the overlap between melatonin and cortisol. If melatonin does not reach its natural peak around 2–3 a.m., the initiation of cortisol production may cause wakefulness around this time.

Melatonin production can be altered for many reasons, such as from working night shifts, light exposure at night, traumatic brain injury, Parkinson disease, aging, dietary factors, or going under general anesthesia. Supplementation with melatonin, an endogenous compound, can be helpful in many circumstances and has been shown safe to use in doses up to 20 mg, although it doesn't take near this dose for most healthy people to get into or help with staying asleep.

The Brain and Sleep: To dig just a bit deeper into the brain, and into how endocannabinoids are helping to modulate sleep, it is necessary to understand the ECS in the homeostasis of neuronal (nerve cells) signaling. The primary homeostatic mechanism of the ECS in neurons is a negative feedback loop for other neurotransmitters signaling.* (See Figure 2.3.)

When a neurotransmitter is released, it is primarily as a result of calcium moving into the cell.** When the neurotransmitter arrives across the divide between neurons (stage 1)—the synaptic space—it binds its receptor and this causes endocannabinoid release upon demand (stage 2). ECBs travel backward as negative feedback loop to the presynaptic neuron, basically to say "got the message." Synaptic transmission is fast and long-distance communication between neurons. The endocannabinoid binds the CB1 receptor on the starting side of the synapse (stage 3) Once the CB1 receptor is engaged, it closes calcium channels which were initially responsible for starting the cascade of releasing the neurotransmitter. If this endocannabinoid homeostasis, or negative feedback loop, is disrupted, the signal keeps feeding forward, resulting in overstimulation of the nerve cells. This is what can happen, for instance, in epilepsy, which is likened to an electrical storm

---

* Neurotransmitters are chemicals released to carry signals from one nerve to another, or to a muscle cell or a gland.

** The membrane separates the inside of the cell from the outside of the cell. Some substances can pass across the double layer of the membrane (either going in or out of the cell) while others must be carried across. This is where proteins that interact with chemical messengers are housed.

in the brain, among other situations associated with hyperactivity in the central nervous system (such as chronic pain, stress, inflammation, or impulsive behaviors).

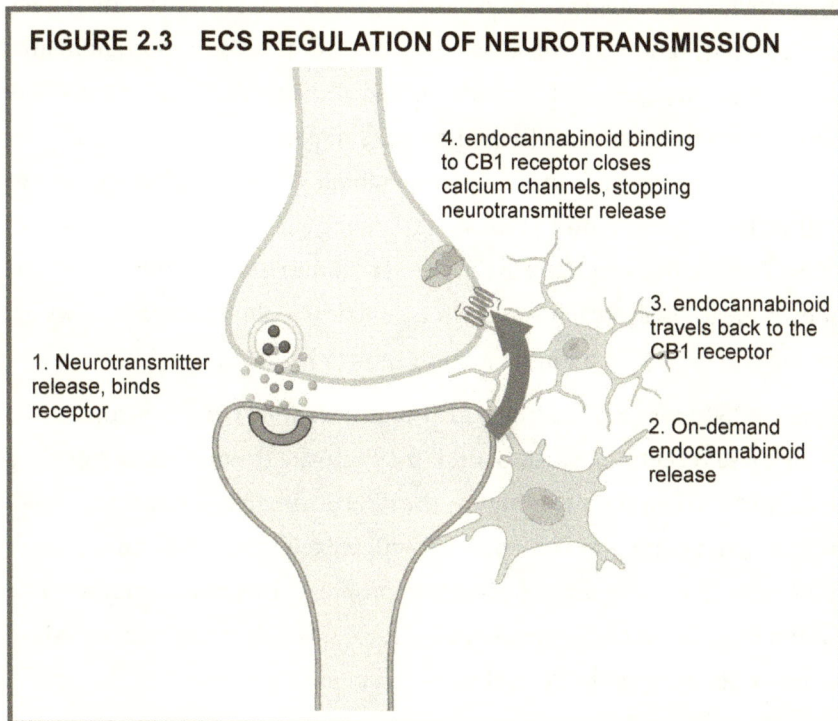

FIGURE 2.3   ECS REGULATION OF NEUROTRANSMISSION

4. endocannabinoid binding to CB1 receptor closes calcium channels, stopping neurotransmitter release

3. endocannabinoid travels back to the CB1 receptor

1. Neurotransmitter release, binds receptor

2. On-demand endocannabinoid release

Most neurotransmitters are stored for release in the neuron; this is a distinction between those other neurotransmitters and the endocannabinoids. This on-demand release is one thing that makes the ECS a homeostatic and unique transmitter system. In Figure 2.3, the two other cells hugging the nerve cells are glia. The spindly one represents a microglia cell, or immune cell in the brain that is always sensing. This cell type is under the control of the CB2R. The other cell is an astrocyte, which also responds to ECS signaling. Both cell types are a communication interface with the nerve cells too, along with the neurotransmitters. These two cells also help in repair, and plasticity of the brain.

In the brainstem is a structure (group of nerve cell bodies) called the pedunculopontine nucleus (PPN) that sends signals to various other parts of the brain. One way that the PPN is involved in sleep is through controlling excitation using the neurotransmitter dopamine for signaling. Remember this neurotransmitter as the one that gives us a reward—feelings of pleasure, satisfaction, and motivation. Another prime neurotransmitter that provides for input is acetylcholine (ACh), a neurotransmitter called the "correlate of human consciousness," one of the most important neurotransmitters in the central nervous system. ACh signals at the space where nerves connect to muscles (telling muscles to contract) and is also key for learning, memory, and attention (more about this in Chapter Forget) as well as for dilating blood vessels and helping glands release their secretions. For our body to make ACh, we need a nutrient, choline, which our body does not make (called an essential nutrient—it is *essential* that we get it from diet- found in highest amounts in meat).

At the PPN, there are nicotinic ACh receptors (that's right, nicotine also binds these receptors); when bound, they activate the dopamine signaling in the PPN. When activity is high in the PPN during the day, there is a lot of ACh signaling going on—associated with wakefulness. This circuit needs to be turned down in order for sleep to progress. This is an important role for the ECS, based on the model in Figure 2.3, which is the homeostasis of neurons signaling in the central nervous system.

There are many connections made between the ECS, cannabis, and acetylcholine. Cannabinoid agonists can both inhibit this release or inhibit acetylcholinesterase (AChE), the enzyme responsible for removing acetylcholine from the nerve clefts—meaning it could go either way, remembering the biphasic concept.

THC has been shown to inhibit AChE, thereby increasing levels of acetylcholine transiently, and may be a means by which it enhances cognitive function. These situations are also biphasic responses, or dose-related, and dose, along with individual biology, determines which direction it may go. Low dose typically provides an increase in ACh (inhibition of AChE) and higher dose inhibits acetylcholine function resulting in anticholinergic responses such as dry mouth, dry eyes, impaired short-term memory, inability to urinate, reduced sweating, and increase in heart rate.

In sleep, the ECS provides a negative feedback loop to prevent ACh from over-activating dopamine neurons in the PPN. This is what is needed at night for sleep—less acetylcholine and less dopamine activity. There are genetic alterations that can keep this from happening, which has been shown in Parkinson's Disease (PD), where there is a loss of the PNP ACh receptors, as well as in schizophrenia and bipolar disorder, where there are genetic changes in sensor allowing for dopamine signaling. Facilitation of the negative feedback of the ECS in this area of the brain could be a key for treating some sleep disorders such as in PD or in some mental health disorders.

One final compound that regulates wakefulness, arousal, and appetite (energy homeostasis) that is affected by the ECS is orexin, found in the brain area of the hypothalamus. The protein receptors for orexin were found to affect NREM sleep and overlap with CBRs. This ECS/orexin interaction includes the joining of these 2 proteins into a form called a heterodimer. When orexin binds its receptors, this induces the synthesis of 2AG, indicating the fundamental negative feedback loop previously described in neurons. This relationship between the orexin system and the ECS involves energy homeostasis, food intake, sleep, arousal and wakefulness.

Cannabinoids and Sleep

Blocking the CB1R (in rats) enhances arousal during their sleep cycle, and in opposition, THC binding or activating CB1R facilitates sleep as a sedative or hypnotic* compound.[69] However, at high dose, THC may disrupt sleep architecture, another example of biphasic effects. Doses of THC between 2–10 mg are recommended; do not go above 10 mg of THC, as this is likely the dose at which disruption of REM sleep starts to occur for many people.[70] THC has also been shown to enhance the release of melatonin in humans who smoked cannabis with a 1% THC potency (so it doesn't take a big dose!). Melatonin peak was 120 minutes after inhaling the cannabis.

---

* Hypnotic means tending to produce sleep. The most common drugs used as hypnotics are benzodiazepines, antidepressants, antipsychotics, antihistamines, and melatonin receptor agonists.

[71] More is not better—there could be a biphasic* effect on melatonin production where high dose of THC inhibits the production of melatonin by the pineal gland.

HERBAN LEGEND #3: Cannabis is equally as bad for sleep as alcohol. This is a stigma about THC and sleep that remains today. However, the biphasic effects on sleep have not been well-studied. Low dose (under 10 mg) has been associated with a strengthening of the ultradian rhythm without disruption of REM sleep.

A 1973 experiment used THC for sleep in people with sleep difficulties at doses of 10, 20, and 30 mg, taken about 1.5 hours prior to regular sleep time for each individual. All 3 doses were observed to shorten the time taken to fall asleep after hitting the pillow and reduce awakenings between midnight and 4 a.m. There were greater side effects at the higher doses and a number of participants reported feeling hung over the next day with 30 mg dose more associated with this effect. At a dose of 17 mg (a single oral dose), REM sleep was measured to be reduced as well as at other high doses (from 61–258 micrograms/kilogram, about a 40 mg starting dose), while other studies have not measured this.

The essential oil component of cannabis can also be of importance when inhaling cannabis for purposes of going to sleep. (See Box 2.1) There is much debate over whether there is any truth to the concept of 2 species of cannabis—C. sativa and C. indica. In a vast amount of cross-breeding, or hybridization of the plant, these distinctions are not recognizable. This distinction was based on the way the plant looked when growing in their natural habitat. Sativa was recognized as tall and spindly with thin leaflets while indica grew closer to the ground with very wide leaflets.

---

* Biphasic means that there can be 2 distinct effects at 2 different doses. This can be easily demonstrated with alcohol intake where at low dose there may be pleasant feelings but with higher doses it is a depressant.

> **HERBAN LEGEND #4:** Cannabis can easily be classified as either sativa or indica. Based on the data from several laboratories the contemporary cannabis found in licensed shops are likely all hybrids and the result of this is a loss of biodiversity of the plant.

What *can* differentiate chemotypes is their essential oil or terpene profile along with other flavor or scent compounds including alcohols, esters and ketones.[72, 73] For a heavy body feeling, myrcene is most likely responsible, and contributions of linalool (found in lavender) or limonene (found in oranges) can also help with relaxation. Linalool has been shown to bind to the same receptor as GABA, our neuroinhibitory neurotransmitter. These compounds are highly bioactive, except after ingestion as when using a cannabis edible. Inhalation (vaporization, not combustion) provides immediate effects of the terpenes while when eaten, the liver changes them before reaching the brain (metabolites). The labeling of oral cannabis as sativa or indica is not always likely to be indicative of whether the products may be more sedating or more stimulating to the body/mind.[74] These effects are prominent when cannabis flower is vaporized (burning combusts the terpenes). You may think you can have the same effects from a vape pen, but typically the essential oil component can be changed by the extraction process and by the high heat of a vape pen. Some manufacturers have used an approach of adding terpenes back in after being lost in the extraction process, but these may not always be the same, or in the identical concentrations and ratios as originally occurring in the plant.

There is not any great evidence that CBD, on its own or taken as an isolate, facilitates sleep. It was demonstrated that CBD, when given at a dose of 400 mg prior to sleep, did not alter or improve sleep architecture.[75] When CBD was injected directly into the hypothalamus of rats, it actually suppressed sleep and caused alertness by increasing the levels of dopamine in the brain![76] However it is known that CBD at higher doses can be sedating and recently this higher dose in combination with terpenes was shown to improve sleep and increase restorative sleep in people with insomnia.[77]

Cannabinol (CBN), a byproduct of the breakdown of THC and thought to be an indicator of cannabis freshness, is being heavily marketed for sleep. There is no solid evidence to support this marketing claim, however.[78] CBN may act similarly to THC at CB1R to facilitate sleep, but it only has about 1/4 the potency at the receptor compared to THC; you would likely need a much higher dose than THC for effectiveness yet it is still unknown if it has the same downstream effects as THC.

> **BOX 2.1 WHAT ARE TERPENES?:** Terpenes are a large class of chemical compounds that can be emitted into the air, known as volatiles, and make up the essential oils of plants. Terpenes are responsible for both smell and flavor characteristics. They are thought to partially modulate differential effects of cannabis chemotypes not the THC or CBD amounts (or the cannabinoid class of compounds). There is wide variability of the essential oil component of cannabis, and some modern research has shown that specific terpenes differentiate distinct chemovars (the breakdown of the plant by its chemical characteristics). Chemovar or chemotype is the formal term (not 'strain'- this is a term used for bacteria) for the different varieties of cannabis in the market place. Despite a wide range of names (and re-naming) or chemovars, Cannabis is a single species but the vast naming scheme misrepresents the actual biodiversity across the chemotypes.

Early studies of THC effects on sleep in humans used high doses, 20–50 mg and 70–210 mg, reporting disruption of REM sleep, with a facilitation of deep sleep at some doses.[79, 80] Recreational doses of THC are capped by many states with regulatory laws at 10 mg, and 5 mg is considered a standard dosing unit as defined by the National Institutes of Health (NIH). The doses used during early research, what many people access now, and what constitutes a therapeutic dose may not be the same and vary across regions of the United States.

> **BOX 2.2 INDICA SATIVA DEBATE:** In a 2014 study, cannabis users from a web-based survey rated indica' as the preference for pain management, sedation and sleep. Sativa was preferred to enhance energy and produce euphoria. This distinction began in the 18th century when botanists noticed two distinct growth structures among plant from different geographic areas of the planet. Those growing between 30-50 degrees latitude shared a short, more bushy appearance with thick production of resin (found as trichomes that hold the cannabinoids and essential oil on the surface of the leaflets). Cannabis plants that have been cultivated for a time typically become hybrids, as growers mixed pollen and flower from different chemotypes and the original chemical composition of a pure species was lost. Most botanical authorities now recognize cannabis as a single highly variable species called Cannabis sativa with the two sub species of sativa and indica. An examination of the diversity across these designations or as a hybrid revealed no distinct difference between those labeled as either indica or sativa!
>
> Vigil, J.M., S.S. Stith, and T. Chanel, Cannabis consumption and prosociality. Sci Rep, 2022. 12(1): p. 8352.
>
> Pearce, D.D., K. Mitsouras, and K.J. Irizarry, Discriminating the effects of Cannabis sativa and Cannabis indica: a web survey of medical cannabis users. J Altern Complement Med, 2014. 20(10): p. 787-91.

People who use cannabis often report that THC improves sleep by helping them get into sleep more quickly, sleeping longer, waking less and feeling more rested in the morning.[81] Does 'indica' cannabis promote sleep better than a hybrid or a sativa? See Box 2.2 for more information about these designations. Better sleep equates to better function during the day, particularly for people with chronic pain, as they will have less daytime pain. For those with inflammation, such as joint pain, autoimmune disease, or cancer, they may feel less creaky or stiff by helping to reduce inflammation in the body/mind. Better sleep will also mean ability to concentrate appropriately and help improve mood (less anxiety, depression).

Inhaled or oral? How to Use Cannabis Most Effectively for Sleep

Taking cannabis orally has a slow onset of effect (taking anywhere from 1–4 hours depending on your GI system), while inhaling cannabis has a rapid effect (within 10–15 minutes). Cannabis vapor (from the flower–please do not smoke or use a vape pen) enters the lungs, moves from the lungs to the blood stream, and gets into the brain with high efficiency (60% bioavailability). Although quick in onset, inhaled cannabis has shorter-lived effects (about 2 hours) while taking cannabis orally can have effects that can extend to 6–8 hours for some people (depending on liver enzymes and genetics). If you want to use cannabis for sleep, oral administration will likely help you sustain sleep better across the night, especially when trying to treat pain that may be disrupting sleep. For some, inhaling cannabis makes them sleepy while for others it can activate the mind to the point that this keeps them from falling asleep. I tend to suggest a fast-acting melatonin (such as a sublingual or dissolved form) for helping to get to sleep (along with good sleep hygiene) or using the inhaled cannabis several hours prior to bedtime to avoid active mind.

Cannabis withdrawal, especially for daily users, has been associated with sleep disturbance and vivid dreaming. Upon withdrawal, heavy cannabis users demonstrated lower total sleep time, decreased slow-wave sleep, and decreased time spent in REM sleep compared to non-cannabis users. This seems to resolve over time, from days to a couple of weeks. When using cannabis for sleep, be aware than you can become habituated to it. If you stop taking it, you can likely expect a few days of vivid dreaming and feeling like you may have slept poorly. The more cannabis you use on a daily basis, the greater the withdrawal effects.

Women and Sleep

Women tend to have a more challenging relationship with sleep than men, starting at an earlier age and with a higher burden of insomnia.[82] How many times have I been on an airplane and a fellow male next to me is out cold within minutes? I might eventually take a little nap, but it takes me an hour to get to sleep and by then the plane is about to land! How many times have I heard any noise inside or outside of the house that awakens me while my male partner is oblivious? Maybe it is a maternal superpower to be easily aroused that helps to ensure survival of an infant that is the culprit. The maternal instinct to "tend and defend" (the female version of fight or flight) keeps us in a state of readiness so we can be awakened more readily.

Women often report more sleep disturbance and poorer sleep quality prior to the menses (from the Latin for month and Greek for moon—the monthly shedding of the uterine lining) compared to the rest of the cycle. The moon time (both menses and the literal full moon) can come with insomnia, disturbing dreams, decreased alertness/concentration, sleepiness, and fatigue. Women's cycles tend to be synchronized to the moon cycle— about 25% of women bleed at the time of the new or full moon. (Moon cycles can also have effects on sleep, such as nighttime wakefulness during a full moon). Artificial light can disrupt these moon/human rhythms, however. Regardless of the lore or science, I prefer "moon time" to the medical term menstruation, so I'll use moon time from now on.

Reproductive Cycling and the ECS

The moon cycle is a rhythmic, continuous parade of events co-occurring between the endocrine system, brain, ovaries, and the uterus. The hypothalamic-pituitary-gonadal (HPG) axis is in charge of reproductive cycling, and as with the HP-GI axis, the ECS is overseeing the activities of this axis.

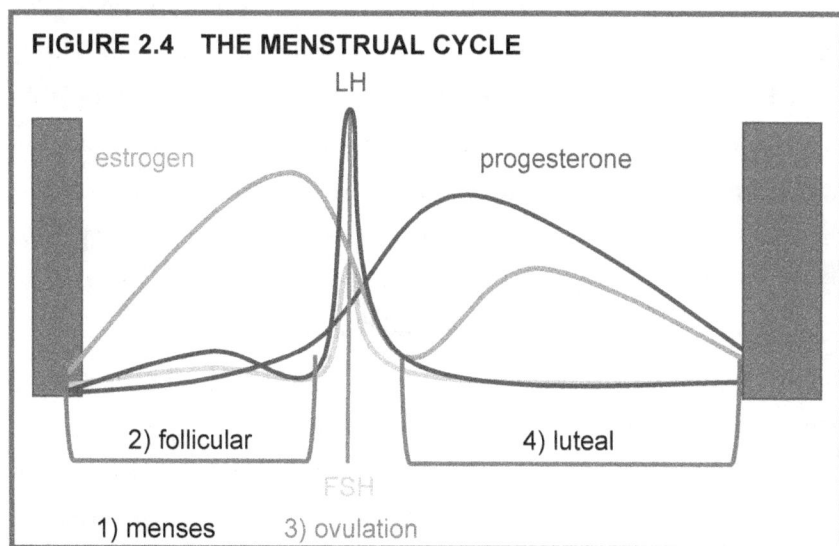

FIGURE 2.4   THE MENSTRUAL CYCLE

LH

estrogen   progesterone

2) follicular   4) luteal

FSH

1) menses   3) ovulation

There have been reports of THC binding to estrogen receptor, but over time this has been disproven. However, THC can modulate steroid hormone pathways, as expected, since the ECS has a role in reproductive tissues. Particularly as we age, estrogen, progesterone, and CBR expression levels are changing; as a result, sleep can become more elusive.

Let's break down the menstrual hormonal cycle: you can use the diagram in Figure 2.4 to help you picture it. There are 4 phases to a full moon cycle: 1) menses (bleeding or shedding of the uterine lining), 2) follicular-rising levels of follicle stimulating hormone (FSH) and the beginning of a surge in estrogen and progesterone, 3) ovulation occurring 1/2–3/4 of the way through the cycle, with a surge of AEA and luteinizing hormone (LH), and 4) luteal—a drop in LH and FSH but rising estrogen and progesterone until the end of the cycle.

The ECS is expressed throughout the reproductive tissues—ovaries, uterus, and fallopian tubes—where it helps regulate the development of egg follicles on the ovaries, maturation of eggs, transport of the egg down the fallopian tube, and implantation of an embryo in the uterus—or not![83] The implantation requires a reduction in AEA levels, as high levels of AEA have been associated with failures of vitro fertilization.[84] The levels of FAAH, the enzyme responsible for degrading AEA, go up at ovulation and this is likely related to the role of the immune system in getting pregnant. Endocannabinoids have been measured in ovaries, follicular fluids, amniotic fluid, and human milk. AEA has been measured in pre-menopausal women, during the early follicular (days 2–6), late follicular (days 8–12), ovulatory (days 13–16), early luteal (days 18–23), and late luteal (days 24–30). It was also measured in pregnant women before and during labor.

Figure 2.5 is representative of how these levels change across the cycle and with age as well as in childbirth (these values were compiled from individual scientific publications[85, 86]). The changes across the cycle are associated with peak levels around the time of ovulation, with AEA levels correlated with FSH and LH, and acting as the negative feedback to bring them back to homeostatic levels.[87] AEA needs to be low for successful implantation of a fertilized egg in the uterus. AEA tends to decrease during the second and third trimesters of pregnancy, and then start to go up until reaching a peak in labor.[88] While AEA levels are not thoroughly understood, it appears they are either controlled by the gonadotropins (compounds that stimulate ovaries and testicles), the sex steroid hormones (estradiol/progesterone), or vice-versa (hormones regulate ECBs).

FIGURE 2.5   ECB LEVELS IN THE MOON CYCLE, LABOR AND MENOPAUSE

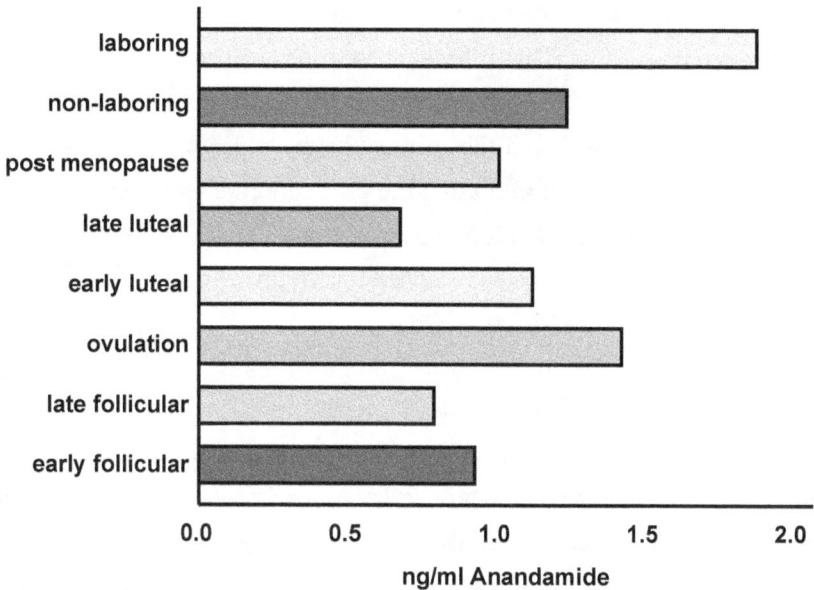

At the initiation of the follicular phase, decreasing activity of the ECS in the hypothalamus (via CB1R) allows for the release of gonadotrophin releasing hormone (GnRH). GnRH then acts on the neighboring pituitary gland telling it to release FSH. FSH does exactly as the name implies: It stimulates tiny follicles (the basic unit on the ovary where the CB1R/CB2R are found), about 10–12 per month (women are born with about 6 to 7-million of these follicles), only one of which will be released as an egg. (In men, FSH stimulates production of sperm.) As the follicles are stimulated, 2 hormones (estradiol and activin) are released by the ovary to enhance FSH production until ovulation occurs. Endocannabinoids then are involved in inhibiting the hypothalamus release of GnRH once it has done its job. THC has also been shown to lower the GnRH concentration in the hypothalamus of female rats, demonstrating the effects of cannabinoids on reproductive homeostasis.

As the follicles mature, the ovary signals back to the pituitary with a compound similar to activin but opposite in action, called inhibin, that starts to *inhibit* the FSH secretion from the pituitary (a negative feedback loop). AEA also spikes and is involved in this negative feedback. The pituitary then releases LH that reaches a peak after 24–48 hours (this is known as a surge) that allows for one follicle that has fully matured to be released from the ovary. (In men, LH stimulates testosterone production). Once an egg has broken out of the follicle, there is a spike in progesterone, made by the mature follicle (from the corpus luteum, a yellow body where the egg emerged), somewhat inhibiting the production of estrogen across the rest of the cycle. The production of progesterone also allows for the uterine lining, the endometrium, to be receptive to a fertilized egg. Progesterone is crucial during the luteal phase.

Hormones and Sleep

These reproductive hormones have a relationship with sleep and circadian function. Estrogen is considered to be a neuroexcitatory hormone. Women with premenstrual depressive disorder (PMDD), which can be due to an imbalance in the estrogen/progesterone/testosterone ratios, have declines in sleep quality, particularly during the late part of the luteal phase. Melatonin has been shown to modulate GABA and the BDNF system in premenstrual syndrome (PMS), which may help with both sleep and mood disorder.[89] Progesterone is considered to be neuroinhibitory, and is needed to counterbalance estrogen-related excitation in the brain. Alternatively, some women with PMDD may report excessive sleep. Studies have found more wakefulness or awakenings during the late luteal phase, and more REM sleep (likely related to a bit higher body temperature after ovulation that is due to the increase in progesterone). Women with polycystic ovarian syndrome (PCOS) who can have an absence of estrogen and progesterone, cycles with no ovulation, and unopposed testosterone may have more sleep disordered breathing that can affect sleep quality.[90]

Our biological rhythm of reproductive hormones, FSH and LH, are also controlled by clock genes. LH is thought to be released at the highest level during the NREM3 sleep phase, illustrating the importance of restorative sleep for fertility and cycling. There are estrogen receptors in the SCN! Short sleep cycles and menstrual cycles are related. While complete understanding of the relationships among sex steroid hormones, sleep, and infertility are still being studied, it is wise to consider that the need to treat the biological clock is likely in order when trying to conceive or when dealing with infertility.[91] In general, consistent sleep periods of less than 6 hours per night may be connected with shorter menstrual cycles.

When taking melatonin orally, the onset of effects is rapid (with a fast-acting form) but our body also metabolizes (the time it takes to leave the system) it quickly. Melatonin is also an important antioxidant and has been shown to peak around the time of ovulation in women. Shift workers (those working night shifts) have longer menstrual cycles, heavier bleeding, and more menstrual pain than those sleeping on a circadian schedule. Melatonin receptors are found on the ovary where it promotes follicle formation and may have a role in treating PCOS. Melatonin is considered to be a safe supplement when trying to conceive.

Should You Take Oral Contraceptives to Help with Sleep?

Combined oral contraceptives (OCs) contain synthetic forms of our natural hormones: ethinyl estradiol and progestin. These are taken for 21 days and then a placebo is taken for 7 days (so that the moon time can occur). During this 21-day administration of synthetic hormones, hypothalamic-pituitary-ovarian (HPO) axis activity is suppressed and your natural of endogenous estradiol and progesterone levels are replaced by the synthetic hormones. While OCs may minimally alter aspects of sleep architecture as well as body temperature, their impact on sleep quality seems to be minimal. Rather than address one element (hormones) that can contribute to sleep difficulties, a systemic approach of treating the whole person will typically bring better and more sustained results, and minimize the need to rely on pharmaceuticals.

I am a strong advocate for NOT using cannabis during pregnancy. There is significant evidence that the ECS has vital roles in the developing brain, and it is not yet fully understood how THC may interfere or disrupt this vital signaling.[92] Additionally, a systematic review and meta-analysis found an association of cannabis use with a greater chance of preterm birth and low birth weight.[93] It is hard to determine if this type of use could be due to smoking or the cannabis itself but other studies suggested an impact on the function of the placenta .

The Change of Life and Sleep

One of the earliest symptoms of women's transition out of the reproductive years is disturbed sleep. This can start to occur in females early in the perimenopause period, long before there is any change in monthly moon-time cycling (which is on average a 21–30-day cycle); the brain is already adapting. This moon time and reproductive transitioning is a neuroendocrine process that eventually results in senescence (from the Latin senex or old), all women undergo it, and it is characterized by stages of transitioning. This is not an illness, but a natural process, just like childbirth.

During this transition out of reproductive years, our major form of estrogen, 17b-estradiol, starts to decline; this is related to the aging of ovaries. This hormonal change sets in motion a broad range of impacts on the brain including changes in glucose metabolism, structural changes, connectivity of brain compartments, and deposits of proteins. Long before a cycling female knows anything is going on, the brain knows. One of the first things to be affected by these silent changes is sleep. This is one of the best times in life for cannabis as an herbal ally. Being beyond the reproductive phase allows for cannabis use without concern for pregnancy, where THC can interfere with the developing brain in the embryo and fetus. Cycling people using cannabis should use birth control and consider discontinuing any cannabis use prior to trying to achieve pregnancy.

Interoceptive Exercise: How do you know when you are sleepy? Do you begin to yawn or just feel drowsy (quiet, peaceful, and relaxed)? Does your body ever feel tired but your brain is not? There are complex relationships between interoception and sleep. Our sensory processes and effects of pain, temperature, habituation, and stressful stimuli can keep us from our sleep.

If you have trouble with sleep, here are some questions to ask yourself:

- Does eating late in the evening stimulate you and keep you awake or does it facilitate falling sleep? Do an experiment and try stopping eating by 6 p.m. or eating a late meal (8 p.m.) and compare results.
- Have you noticed an effect between your temperature and feeling sleepy? Both intense heat and cold exposure close to bedtime can impede sleep. Try taking a warm bath (best with two pounds of Epsom salts) and see how it affects sleepiness. Melatonin is thermoregulatory, so you can try using a small dose (1–3 mg) to experiment how this affects your sleep efficiency.
- Our interoceptive sensitivity should decrease at night to protect our sleep and minimize arousal. Is your sleeping space sacred for you? Is it the right temperature, noise level, and darkness level to facilitate rest?
- If you have any type of chronic pain, keep a diary of your daily sleep and experience of pain. Your pain threshold may be lowered by not getting adequate sleep.
- If you have a bad night of sleep, notice if there is any effect on your hunger the next day.
- Overall, a better night of sleep is associated with fewer concerns about health and less awareness of body pain, while insomnia enhances awareness of pain.
- Do you snore or have apnea? If you think you might, use a sleep tracker or get a formal sleep test.

Disrupted Sleep

Insomnia: Insomnia is defined as too much waking, a problem more than 1/3 of people may struggle with. Short-term insomnia is defined as occurring for <3 months vs. long-term insomnia, which is more than 3 nights per week for >3 months. Insomnia is associated with chronic pain, intake of substances that disturb sleep (alcohol, nicotine, caffeine), chronic stress, anxiety, and some other serious health issues such as traumatic brain injury and cancer.

Restless Leg Syndrome (RLS): RLS is an uncomfortable, and for some an uncontrollable, urge to move your legs and feet—most commonly occurring in the late afternoon to early evening and/or at night. This urge is also accompanied by abnormal sensations such as throbbing, itching, crawling, or aching that is relieved by moving the legs. What causes RLS is not completely understood, but iron deficiency can be one cause, along with alterations in dopamine signaling, which is associated with abnormal movements. RLS symptoms decrease with drugs that stimulate the dopamine system; RLS symptoms can be caused by decreased dopamine signaling or by blocking this signaling in the brain. Because dopamine levels are low in the afternoon, this could correlate with the timing that many patients report for the starting of RLS symptoms. Another theory is that there is impaired oxygenation of tissues due to poor blood flow. For some patients with severe RLS, inhalation of cannabis (through vaporization of flower) can be helpful and even help eliminate it altogether. Hot baths with magnesium sulfate (Epsom salts) can help to relax muscles (use 2 pounds in a full tub of hot water for 20 minutes). Some non-opioid pain relievers have been shown to help. I use lithium orotate clinically for this along with inhaled or oral cannabis. Dosage of THC has not been studied so the optimal dose is unknown, but some people report reduction or remission of symptoms. CBD was not found to be helpful for RLS at doses ranging from 75-300 mg.[94]

Sleep Apnea: If you have ever had the experience of waking up feeling short of breath, you may have experienced sleep apnea. Snoring is often associated with apnea, so if you sleep with someone, ask if they ever hear you snoring. This is among the most common of sleep disorders (overall experienced more by men than women). Undiagnosed sleep apnea, which is thought to occur 80% of the time, can contribute to poor sleep quality and affect health, specifically high blood pressure, heart disease, stroke risk, and risk of cognitive dysfunction. Other symptoms can include headache in the morning, extreme fatigue, brain fog, difficulty concentrating, and irritability.

There are two types of apnea: obstructive and central. Obstructive sleep apnea (OSA) can be due to sleeping on your back, being overweight, having sinus or nasal congestion, or anatomical features. After women go through menopause, the relaxation of tissues due to loss of estrogen could cause or compound this. Central sleep apnea (CSA) is a failure at the level of the brain to regulate gas exchange. CSA can be caused in high altitudes as well as be associated with obesity and with chronic use of narcotics, such as opioids. An overnight sleep study (this can be done at home) can help to diagnose whether you may have sleep apnea. The most common treatment is to use a positive pressure device, known as a continuous positive airway pressure (CPAP) device. These can be highly effective, but many patients despise having to wear them. There have been two studies of THC for decreasing the apneic index (how much apnea is occurring) showing that synthetic THC (dronabinol/Marinol) may help decrease the apneic index (amount of apnea) and strengthen ultradian rhythms.[95, 96] Both of the studies were in OSA, but substituting cannabis (with THC) for opioids may also help to improve CSA.

Sleep Behavior Disorders (SBD): SBD can include sleepwalking, sleep talking, acting out of dreams (known as parasomnias), and occur during REM where there is a loss of the paralysis that occurs during REM. It is thought to occur in about 2% of people, but is under-recognized. The severity can range from mild to violent and may be recognized first by a bed partner who has been injured or moved to another room to sleep. This condition is widespread in people with PD, multiple system atrophy, and dementia with Lewy bodies. Both males and females can have SBD, but males are much more likely to experience and to have more violent episodes than females.

Half of patients with RBD develop RBD after starting an antidepressant medication, and is more prevalent in younger vs. older persons.

This is an important condition to recognize and have diagnosed as there is an association between SBD and cognitive health. Diagnosis and early treatment are critical to avoid cognitive impairment, or more rapid cognitive impairment as in the case of PD. Using a protocol that employs both short- and long-acting melatonin with THC at bedtime has been helpful in my clinical practice. I have worked with many patients with PD who report significant improvement in their sleep using this protocol. Because melatonin is rapidly metabolized, a sustained-release formula is often needed, in addition to a short-acting form. Melatonin seems to be tolerated well and may help to suppress SBD in the majority of patients (6–18 mg). CBD was not found to be helpful for sleep behavior disorder at doses of 75-300 mg.[ ] Of course, optimizing circadian timing of sleep and following general sleep hygiene are important. Avoiding anticholinergic agents (acetylcholinesterase inhibitors), benzodiazepines, and antihistamines is suggested as these agents have been reported to contribute to cognitive dysfunction. (More on this class of drugs in Relax.)

Nightmares and Night Terrors: Nightmares are REM-related phenomena consisting of disturbing mentation and recalled in vivid detail. Nightmares are often characterized by sleep paralysis, an inability to move, defend oneself, or scream. Unlike nightmares, a person having a night terror does not wake up, but while asleep can exhibit intense fear, flailing, and screaming. Night terrors affect more children than adults and typically they will not remember the event the next day. The most common age is 1.5 years, up to 13 years, and can occur at least once in about half of all children.

Nightmares often accompany a diagnosis of PTSD; the two are intertwined. Those who have nightmares have more severe PTSD symptoms, and the nightmares can persist across the lifetime, while the PTSD symptoms can fade. A recent study of medical cannabis patients showed that they had fewer awakenings, and using cannabis just prior to sleep may help decrease awakenings or a lower likelihood of experiencing nightmares.[97] When PTSD is severe in nature, antipsychotics can help to provide some stabilization in the short term. For help with recovering from PTSD, an integrative approach using psychotherapy transcranial magnetic stimulation, ketamine therapy, and/or psychedelics could also be explored.

Naturopathic/Integrative/Functional Approaches

Care of the ECS: Try this breathing trick to help you fall asleep: Breathe in through your nose for 4 seconds, hold your breath for 7 seconds, and exhale through your mouth for 8 seconds; repeat 3 times. Try massage and skin-to-skin cuddling or spooning. Skin contact is an essential nutrient and results in ECB release and elevates oxytocin—both calming chemicals! And oxytocin leads to more ECB release. Mild stretching before bedtime can facilitate release of anti-inflammatory compounds and promote relaxation along with release of ECBs. Orgasm has been shown to release 2AG; this includes orgasm with masturbation.[98]

Terpene: Myrcene: Myrcene is a compound found in many aromatic plants including cannabis, hops, parsley, rosemary, and 200 other plants. It was shown to increase sleep time in rats, and is thought to provide sedating effects in cannabis chemotypes that are dominant in myrcene. This could be what, in part, could comprise an indica type of plant by influencing subjective effects of feeling a heavy body, couch lock, or sedation.[99] These sedative effects may thereby help to initiate sleep or improve sleep. A small study gave myrcene in a capsule form (oral) and reported that on a driving test this compound impaired driving, implicating it as having a sedative effect.[100]

Measuring Allostatic Load: You can measure your AL by across-the day collection of saliva samples (4 samples)—cortisol may be elevated late in the day with sleep disturbance, circadian disruptions and altered HPA axis; urine tests that measure the breakdown of catecholamines (epinephrine and norepinephrine—there are specialty labs that do this); insulin; blood pressure (hypertension); inflammatory cytokines; C-reactive protein, a non-specific marker of inflammation cardiovascular disease along with F_2isoprostanes, total cholesterol, homocysteine; and thyroid function tests.

Herbal Allies

Valeriana officinalis: Valerian has a long history of use as a sedative and grows all over the world. The essential oil (2%) of this plant is distinct, with some describing it as smelling of dirty socks. It is one of nature's most powerful muscle relaxers too. It has been described to contain GABA, a neuroinhibitory transmitter, to facilitate the release of GABA or inhibit the breakdown. Valerian has also been shown to reduce blood pressure and heart rate. This slowing of central nervous system activity may be why it has been found to have a significant effect on improved sleep. Be aware that some people can have a paradoxical reaction to valerian and have an anxious and restless feeling. You may want to try it first during the day. It is best if used in a standardized extract containing valerenic acids.

Scutellaria laterifolia: Skullcap typically grows in woods and meadows, native to the Eastern US and is another traditional sedative that is a member of the mint family. This herbal ally may be better used for relaxation of anxiety, also action through GABA channels, and by acting on anxiety may help with insomnia. It is often used in combination with other sedating herbs. There is not good evidence that it alone will significantly affect sleep.

Matricaria chamomilla: Chamomile is a well-known and loved plant that is a member of the daisy family and grows wild all over the world. It contains many interesting constituents and has been used widely all over the world as a medicine (including for treatment of stomach problems). The terpenoid alpha bisabolol (a sesquiterpene), also found in some cannabis, has been an important indicator of its potency (good for wound healing and skin problems). Chamomile tea is among the world's most popular teas and has been valued as a mild tranquilizer with hypnotic activity (probably also through GABA) calming nerves and reducing anxiety, nightmares, insomnia, and other sleep problems. Try a cup an hour or so before bedtime. Some people are allergic to this family of plants, but this is usually when used on the skin.

Passiflora incarnata: Purple passionflower is a lovely vine native to the Southeastern/Eastern US as well as Central and South America that will take over your garden! The unusual and beautiful flower is the source of anxiolytic and sedative actions, used by Native Americans to treat insomnia and nervousness, with a good safety profile. It is a nervine (nerve tonic) and may have analgesic and antispasmodic effects. A flavonoid, apigenin, and chrysin may be the compounds that could help with sleep, again acting through GABA receptors or modulating reuptake of GABA. One study in humans used 1500 mg of an extract, and another used 3 cups of tea per day.

Piper methysticum: Kava kava is a member of the pepper family that is a vine used ceremonially in its native Pacific Islands. Yangonin is a member of a compound family called kavalactones that has been shown to bind to cannabinoid receptors and also to potentiate GABA receptors. It is known for relaxing and enhancement of well-being. It's wise to be judicious with this plant as some preparations have been reported to induce liver damage. Root extracts standardized for kavalactones are probably going to be the most effective for helping relax you for sleep.

Supplements: Melatonin is the most commonly used supplement for sleep. Doses of a fast-acting form of 1–5 mg can be helpful for falling asleep, while sustained-release forms are more helpful for those needing help staying asleep. (Lithium orotate may help with circadian dysfunction and this is discussed further in Forget.) Some people use 5HTP, the precursor for serotonin, but there is no guarantee that the 5HTP will convert to melatonin. It is more likely to be transformed to serotonin by gut bacteria and used locally in the gut. By taking epigallocatechin gallate (EGCG- a compound from green tea) along with 5HTP it may be possible to prevent the conversion of 5HTP to serotonin in the gut. It was shown to be helpful in people with PD who suffered from sleep behavior disorder (50 mg).[101] 5HTP was also found useful for children suffering from night terrors (2 mg/kg at bedtime).[102] For women who have PCOS or estrogen dominance, supplementing with oral micronized progesterone can be helpful in some instances. For helping the mind to relax magnesium threonate, a form thought to more easily cross over into the brain, as a co-factor for serotonin production and acting on GABA receptors, the brain's calming neurotransmitter.

Food/Nutrition: There are some foods that are thought to be rich in melatonin or promote the synthesis of it. Tart cherries have been reported to be one source and milk, a traditional remedy for insomnia, may also be high in melatonin. Nuts and eggs as well as foods high in tryptophan (the amino acid that is the precursor for making serotonin and melatonin) found in oats, bananas, turkey, chicken, milk, cheese, and chocolate (highest in milk and turkey). Cofactors for helping the biosynthesis of melatonin include iron, folate, zinc, B6 magnesium, and vitamin C.

The time across the day that we eat should be synchronized with our circadian rhythms. Eating late in the evening, prior to bedtime, or eating for more hours of the day, leads to metabolic dysfunction. Time-restricted eating (intermittent fasting) has been shown to increase the duration of sleep and reduce apnea. It may also help to lower insulin levels and increase melatonin. Weight gain can be kept to a minimum by simply restricting eating to an 8–12-hour window in the day. This time-restricted eating schedule may not directly impact sleep architecture, but by helping to reduce obesity may impact snoring or sleep apnea and thereby improve overall sleep quality and health.

Basics of Good Sleep Hygiene

- Try to get your exercise early in the day (at least 20 minutes).
- Get daily sunlight exposure.
- Develop a bedtime routine—winding down, hot bath or shower, reading, cuddling.
- Sleep environment should be restful (dark, quiet, temp, noise). Avoiding stimulation 30 minutes prior to sleep by limiting blue-light exposure, doing an enjoyable task (take a bath, listening to relaxation music, podcast, or instruction on mindfulness).
- Try to avoid reading or watching TV in bed—make the bedroom a sacred space for sleeping.
- Regulate your sleep/wake times: establish regular bedtime, prior to midnight.
- Use relaxation exercises prior to sleep (such as deep abdominal breathing) or listening to music with a slow tempo, similar to heart rate (80 beats per second).
- Avoid daytime napping.

- Avoid drinking alcohol—alcohol is metabolized to an aldehyde that can lead to wakefulness in the middle of the night (and hangover during the day).
- Don't eat a heavy meal or consume caffeine after 6 p.m. Some slow metabolizers of caffeine may need to stop any consumption after noon (lunch time).

Yoga/Chakras: The sixth chakra, Ajna, means to command. The color associated with this chakra is deep indigo, symbolizing purification. It is located just above the eyebrows between the eyes, often called the third eye, and associated with the pineal gland. It is connected to our nightmares, emotional hypersensitivity, memory, and lack of clarity. To engage this chakra is to enter a multidimensional vision. We engage this when in self-introspection (seeing into our feelings, objectively), balancing our higher self with the body. Practices such as journaling, meditating, Jungian psychotherapy, stargazing, and prayerful expressions are practices that open this chakra. Getting into nature and out into the sunlight every day is important for ajna. Balasana is known as child's pose and is one of the most effective for calming the central nervous system (CNS). It can help to improve circulation and normalize the breath to ready yourself for bed. Bhramari pranayam, or humming bee, is a pranayama that can help to harness your energy from the day and prepare the nervous system for sleep. Headstand is a yoga pose associated with this chakra.

Monitoring Cannabis Effects on Sleep

Trials	Date/ Time	Oral/ Inhaled	Dose/ Product	Total Hours Asleep	# Times Awake	Dreaming Y/N	Time to Fall Asleep	Refreshed Y/N
1								
2								
3								
4								

CHAPTER 3

Relax

> *"If you are distressed by anything external, the pain is not due to the thing itself, but to your estimate of it; and this you have the power to revoke at any moment"* —Marcus Aurelius, Roman emperor

Overview

I am gliding on my bicycle, downhill from my house toward the beach. With each block, I can feel the temperature dropping a degree or two due to the cool temperature of the ocean. As I get closer, I can see the surface texture of the water. Is the water glassy today? I notice the color of the ocean, which ranges from deep blue to turquoise depending on the time of year, water temperature and wind conditions. I am picking up the smell and taste of the salty air more distinctly the nearer I am to the sand and sea. I start to hear the breaking of the waves, today close to the shore and more diffuse than on days with big waves. It is a relaxing white noise that starts to permeate my soul. The seagulls are calling overhead. I park my bike and take off for the sand, feeling the grains between my toes, my feet sinking comfortably into the collected warmth. I stand and take in deep gulps of ocean air, inviting the ocean microbiome to invade my lungs. In minutes, I am transformed by the beauty and rejuvenating power of nature.

The Stress Response

Have you ever noticed that you had a stress response that left you feeling drained, debilitated, anxious, sleepless, or depressed? The ability to recognize and acknowledge that a situation has become difficult or painful, *and* the ability to choose a different response leading to peace rather than turmoil, is known as stress resilience. This resilience is enhanced by honing interoception. In a nutshell, the more stress you are exposed to in your lifetime, the more your resilience to stress can be impaired. If stress affected your mother when she was pregnant with you, or if you experienced chronic stress during your childhood, the physical and mental effects can be pronounced and long lasting. Stress adds up over our lifetime culminating not only from present-time stressors, but also effects of stressors that may have begun when you were in the womb. You can still carry the stress your mother was experiencing, and her mother before her—this ancestral stress is a part of your biochemical make-up.

Although fear and anxiety are normal emotions, they can become detrimental to health in many ways, particularly if a stress response is triggered over and over again or when the triggers are extreme in intensity and/or duration. When ongoing, untreated, or unaddressed, a continual activation of our stress responses affects life and health in negative ways. These effects are primarily on the hypothalamic-pituitary-adrenal (HPA) axis, the connection between the brain and adrenal glands. Adrenal glands sit on top of each of your kidneys and regulate not only the stress response, but also metabolism, blood pressure, immune and kidney function.

Thinking across your life, what is the earliest threat, fear, scary experience, fright, terror, or any kind of conflict that you can remember experiencing or having directed toward you? It could be anything across a wide spectrum, from getting lost in a store to being physically abused. Nothing is too small to remember or to count as a potential traumatic experience. One of my early memories is of abandonment at age 5 when my mother dropped me off at church for a vacation bible school. She refused to walk me in, even though I really wanted that (I was an extremely shy child), and insisted that I walk in with my older siblings. As she drove off, we entered the building and my siblings were told that my kindergarten class was not starting until the next day: there was no class for me that day. I begged to go to the second-grade class with my sister, but "they" refused to allow this and sent me to stay in the nursery with the babies until my mom came to pick us up. I was humiliated, anxious, felt abandoned and vividly remember sitting in the corner with my hands over my face until my mother came for me hours later. This is still a striking memory for me and an example of how stressful events for a child don't necessarily have to be extreme trauma (known as capital-T trauma) like exposure to physical abuse, extreme neglect or gun or other violence.

Body/Mind Interface #3

I want you to take a few deep breaths then close your eyes. Your task is to see your childhood self when you were in a happy, contented, or safe environment that you experienced as a child. Allow yourself to see the space, taking the time to take in any colors, smells, other people present, sounds, and anything else about the environment. Take about 5 minutes and allow yourself to be immersed in the experience. What is your small-self doing here? Why are they there? Approach your small self in this place and gently give them a hug. Tell them that you will protect them and you want them to come on a journey with you. Take their hand and walk together out of the space and into the sunlight.

Were you able to connect with your small self? Did you have any experience of what you may have felt at that time in life? What is your experience now around that time of your life?

The Physiology of Stress

The common bodily responses to danger, or the fight-or-flight response, (or for women the tend-and-defend/befriend response: see Box 3.1) includes an increase in heart rate, dilating of the pupils, dry mouth, faster breathing or breathlessness, freezing (not being able to move), sweating, and sometimes needing to move the bowels. The flash flood of stress hormones responsible for these physiologic responses and associated feelings includes epinephrine (or adrenaline, the first hormone to activate the brain) and then a surge of cortisol that follows the epinephrine. Both stress hormones are made in the adrenal glands.

> **BOX 3.1   TEND AND DEFEND/BEFRIEND:** Evolutionary biology has suggested that females may have evolved differently from males in their response to stress. Observations have revealed that affiliating with other humans under conditions of threat help to ensure survival of offspring for protection and survival. This stress response may be more focused on release of oxytocin and endogenous opioid compounds. This response is thought to be an alternative to an aggressive or antagonistic reaction to a threat. Either way, the biological systems help to mobilize the body to rise to the demand of a threatening encounter and then return to homeostasis. Tending includes nurturing one another and building social connections.
>
> *Taylor, S.E., et al., Biobehavioral responses to stress in females: tend-and-befriend, not fight-or-flight. Psychol Rev, 2000. 107(3): p. 411-29.*

The next step in this biochemical response is that cortisol travels to many places in the body. One of these places is back to the brain where it helps tell your body that danger has passed. As children we were likely not very aware of, or in tune with, this bodily response, and did not know what it meant, how to interpret it, or how to manage it. Unfortunately, it is likely that many of us were not instructed as children how to recognize and name any feelings including anxiety, fear, or panic. We also probably weren't taught how to manage those feeling with tools like bringing the feeling to conscious awareness or to simply slow our breathing. Many of us did not receive any comfort in such a situation. Rather, we were sent on our way with the impact of trauma on our body and psyche becoming normalized and integrated into our being. We coped and developed adaptive mechanisms because our brain was trained that this was normal.

Stress-related disorders are one of the most prevalent healthcare problems plaguing society, affecting over 30% of adults in the US, and even more highly prevalent in adolescents. Examples of these disorders include generalized anxiety disorder (GAD), social anxiety disorder, panic disorder, separation anxiety, and PTSD. Characteristic of these stress-related adaptations is excessive fear, catastrophizing, and the attempt to avoid anything that could trigger anxiety. And this does not include the physical health implications of the allostatic load that can cause chronic health problems. You can use the app to assess yourself.

If you lived in an environment where there was repeated stress your body responded by adapting to this stress in a process called allostasis. Over time, allostasis results in a deficiency in cortisol levels. When this occurs, the negative feedback loop signal provided by cortisol—which should bring the HPA axis, associated neurotransmitter levels, and pro-inflammatory molecules back to baseline or homeostasis— becomes impaired. As a result of this malfunction, inflammation is allowed to creep into the body. The resulting inflammation affects not only physical but also emotional *and* mental health. But the loop is not broken beyond repair! It is this repair that I hope you will learn about and develop tools for with this book as your guide.

Minimizing and managing the stress in our life is foundational for health, well-being, and key for avoiding disease. Efficient and effective treatments for stress-related disorders such as anxiety disorders are major challenges in healthcare and medicine. This chapter will inform you about ways that you can work to help restore and maintain your stress resilience by helping the body come back to its set point (homeostasis). A prime goal is to increase your ability to rise to a stressful event in a healthy way.

Sometimes it's hard to embark on any kind of activity, goal-oriented or not, when suffering from chronic anxiety. Chronic anxiety (eg, worrying excessively about normal everyday situations, irritability, difficulty concentrating, and a host of physical symptoms) is debilitating in many ways. It can rob us of friendships, professional development, energy to complete simple tasks, appropriate sleep, and cause physical unwellness. If any of these things describe you, the best thing you can do for yourself is to develop a relationship with a qualified therapist right away! There are many types of therapy that can help you navigate difficult emotions and techniques to help you tame and overcome fear and anxiety, thus helping to restore your body/mind health.

The ECS is an important mediator of the physiological response to stress. A lot of people who use cannabis for medical benefit report that anxiety is the number 2 reason they use cannabis (pain is number 1).[103] People who use cannabis for anxiety also report that they may decrease the use of antianxiety prescription medications.[104] One reason that people report cannabis helping with anxiety is because THC acts directly on the ECS, activating both the CB1R and CB2R as our body's endocannabinoids do. There is an important distinction however—THC is much more potent than our body-made cannabinoids. The ECS is a key for modifying the stress response and while THC can be a hack for anxiety (or it can exacerbate anxiety), recovering and building your resilience is the ultimate goal. How do you go about doing this? Through a step-by-step process that can be likened to swimming upstream! The point is to get to the root cause, address and then build health.

Using Cannabis for Anxiety or Stress Reduction

Some cannabis users report reduction in anxiety symptoms shortly after using cannabis.[105] Low doses of THC have been shown to be anxiolytic (or reduces anxiety) while increasing THC doses can induce anxiety.[106] THC can be a good hack for anxiety, but is not a fix for the underlying cause. Getting too high of a dose of THC can cause anxiety, increase social anxiety, induce paranoia, and rarely even an episode of psychosis.[107, 108] With cannabis now super-potent and products on the market with super high doses, it can appear normal to use such high-potency cannabis. In fact, these super-potency products are almost purified drugs and may not resemble the plant at all! Toning the ECS with low dose THC is the best approach. Especially for people with trauma, where the CB1R may be downregulated, tolerance can be low and first CBR receptor levels need to be upregulated.

Individuals can respond to the same dose of cannabis in different ways, so starting with milli- to microdosing (low sub-milligram doses of THC) is a strategy. Because of these biphasic effects of THC on anxiety, erring on the side of caution is best, going with low dose until you know how it hits you. Other factors that could impact how you react to cannabis are your

Time for a Body Connection Check-in:

First place yourself on the line.

←——————————————————————————————→

++Body Awareness   **Body Detachment++**

For each statement below, assess yourself on this scale: not at all, a little bit, sometimes, most of the time, all of the time.

_____ 1. If there is tension in my body, I am aware of the tension.

_____ 2. I feel like I am looking at my body from outside of my body.

_____ 3. I take cues from my body to help me understand how I feel.

_____ 4. I can feel my breath travel through my body when I exhale deeply.

_____ 5. I distract myself from feelings of physical discomfort.

For each time you answered not at all, score a zero; a little bit = 1; some of the time = 2; most of the time = 3; and all of the time = 4. These questions are part of a larger survey on the Scale of Body Connection. How do you score? Statements 1, 3, and 4 assess your body connection so a higher score is better. Statements 2 and 5 assess your body dissociation, so a lower score is better. Place a mark on the line where you rate yourself and compare this to the second rating that you performed in the Sleep chapter.

individual biochemistry, the setting in which you use cannabis, or your expectations about THC. Understanding how to use THC wisely is important. A low-potency cannabis (3%–10% THC) flower vaporized (even one brief inhalation) can provide immediate effects and be a hack for some people. Similarly, 1–2 mg of THC is probably enough for many people when taking it orally. To tone ECS function a microdose of 0.5 mg is suggested.

CBD has also been tried for anxiety but the effective dose from research is in the hundreds of milligrams, making this a potentially unaffordable prospect for long-term use. CBD is not directly impacting the ECS as THC does, and it is unclear exactly how CBD may work in anxiety, but has been shown to activate serotonin receptors. This is the proposed mechanism for antidepressant drugs, which are often prescribed for anxiety (selective serotonin reuptake inhibitors: SSRI). Using CBD in a preparation that such as a full-spectrum hemp product can be a low THC approach. Using a 25:1 ratio of CBD to THC may provide gentle benefit from both compounds, along with the full spectrum of cannabinoids in the whole plant (see Box 3.2).

The essential oil component of cannabis flower also contributes to the overall effects of cannabis, most notable and bioavailable when inhaled and when cannabis flower is vaporized. The terpenes that may promote calming effects and relaxation are linalool, myrcene, and beta-caryophyllene. Linalool is found in lavender and can bind the GABA receptor, producing anxiolysis. [109] Beta-myrcene has been shown to have sedative effects; you may have experienced its calming effects with cannabis's cousin plant hops (*humulus lupulus*).[110] Beta-caryophyllene is a scent you would recognize, found in abundance in cloves and black pepper. This terpene is a dietary cannabinoid and has been shown to activate CB2R receptor, but not CB1R.[111] Activating CB2R results in downregulation of inflammation, and can affect anxiety (since inflammation and anxiety are closely intertwined).

The ECS Provides That We Relax

At the deepest and more primitive levels of your brain, the ECS is active. CB1Rs are heavily implicated in modulating our stress responsiveness, along with the endocannabinoids AEA and 2AG. CB1 is found in large numbers in brain areas involved in keeping our emotional responses in check: the hippocampus, hypothalamus, and amygdala. These receptors and the endocannabinoid lipid transmitters modulate the HPA axis. The ECS is a primitive system and is one of the early interfaces between the neuro (brain) and endocrine (hormonal) systems (neuroendocrine) beginning with our development in the womb.

> **BOX 3.2 TYPES OF HEMP PRODUCTS:** Hemp is cannabis. By the definition of our United State Federal government, the cannabis must contain <0.3% THC to be considered hemp. The US Farm Bill in 2018 legalized growing of hemp for agricultural purposes, an important fiber crop. However, this legalization did not specifically set regulations for extraction of the phytochemicals, namely the chief component cannabidiol (CBD), to sell as a nutritional supplement.
>
> The one exception is the FDA-approved drug, *Epidiolex*, that is a purified, pharmaceutical grade isolate of CBD. Both cannabis and hemp products including CBD are not considered to be regulated under the current framework for other supplements. Despite this, there is a plethora of CBD or hemp products being marketed and sold.
>
> The terms full spectrum, broad spectrum, isolate, and minor cannabinoids are used.
>
> - Full spectrum is a whole plant hemp extract that will contain THC.
> - Broad spectrum is a whole plant extract from which THC has been purged.
> - An isolate is when a single molecule has been isolated and the other cannabis compounds are not present.
> - Minor cannabinoids are those that exist in a very low level in the plant but are now being exploited.
> - Minor cannabinoids include cannabigerol (CBG), cannabichromene (CBC), tetrahydrocannabivarin (THCV), acid cannabinoids (which are unstable and convert to other compounds), and others.

Anatomy of the Stress Response

What happens when you feel stress is generated in part by the ECS. The response begins when you sense danger (seeing, hearing, smelling) and the sympathetic nervous system secretes adrenaline. This burst of adrenaline circulates rapidly through the body causing the heart to beat faster, dilating blood vessels, pupils, and airways, and increasing blood pressure. These things to allow us to run away fast by delivering more blood to our muscles and more oxygen through our blood. Our sight, hearing, and other senses become sharpened and all of this happens so quickly that we are not aware that it is happening.

This entire cascade (known as the sympathetic or autonomic [automatic] nervous system response) occurs before we have the chance to fully process what is happening visually or cognitively. After this adrenaline burst, there is a short-term rise in the level of 2AG in the brain, specifically in the amygdala and prefrontal cortex (where our higher-level thinking occurs). The higher the 2AG level, the more likely we are to experience freezing—trying to be still and quiet until danger passes. You have probably had this happen before. Acetylcholine (Ach) is another neurotransmitter involved in this automatic response, as a defensive neurochemical response to threat. Threat-induced freezing is a neurobiological mechanism, a state of attentive immobility, and likely occurs to put a brake the sympathetic system. This brake provides us with the opportunity to enhance our perception or awareness of what is happening as a preparation for taking action against the threat. Enhanced perception is an effect of THC, similar to what 2AG may be doing in this instance.

The temporary rise in 2AG (see 1. in Figure 3.1) serves to reduce the levels of anandamide in the hypothalamus. The purpose of anandamide is to regulate the HPA. AEA is normally responsible for inhibiting or slowing down our emotional responses to stress: worry, fear, and panic (thus the bliss). But in this instance of acute stress, the decrease in anandamide provides a feed-forward mechanism for the HPA axis (2.). It promotes the secretion of cortisol from the adrenal glands by allowing for corticotropin-releasing hormone (CHR) to be released by the hypothalamus. The CHR then signals the pituitary to release adreno-corticotropic hormone, which travels in the blood stream to the adrenal glands. Then the adrenal glands increase cortisol production (3.) as well as production of other steroid molecules (aldosterone and androgens). This increase in cortisol is intended to occur in the short term (a normal part of mounting the stress response). The normal production of cortisol should provide a negative feedback loop to the brain. When cortisol then travels through the bloodstream and reaches the brain, this is a signal for anandamide levels to go back up. Typically, this feedback loop should happen within 10 minutes of cortisol being released (if your stress resilience is working). When AEA goes up in the hypothalamus, the signal for the adrenal glands to produce cortisol is turned down. The ECS is working to bring you back into balance, biochemically in the process known as homeostasis.

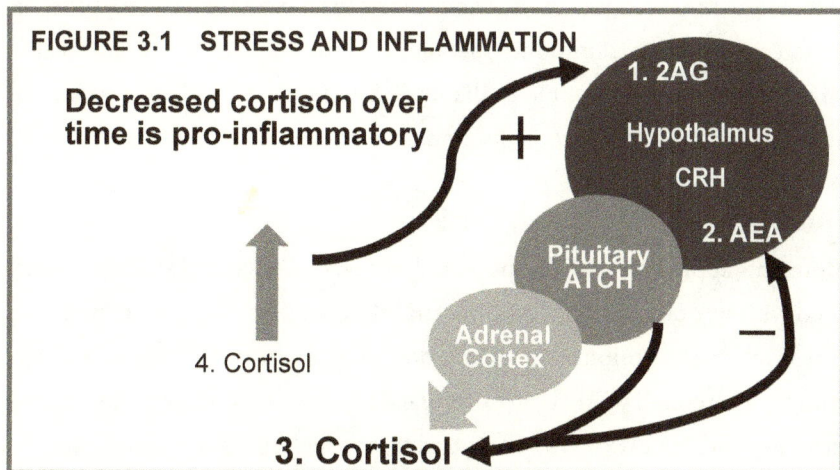

FIGURE 3.1 STRESS AND INFLAMMATION

Decreased cortison over time is pro-inflammatory

1. 2AG
Hypothalamus
CRH
2. AEA

Pituitary
ATCH

Adrenal
Cortex

4. Cortisol

3. Cortisol

Outside of the brain however, AEA levels in the blood have been measured and found to be elevated during short-term stress. For example, there are studies where acute social stress and motion sickness led to increased anandamide levels in the bloodstream.[112] The higher someone's AEA level was at baseline (prior to the stressor), the less stress they reported. AEA in the blood may be a yet unproven biomarker for acute stress. It has been hypothesized that AEA is elevated in the beginning of a stress cycle or at the initiation of stress, but may be depleted over time, in the situation of chronic stress. Once stress becomes chronic or continues over a long period of time, then 2AG becomes elevated in the blood, indicating that 2AG could then be a biomarker for long-term stress.[113] The effects of stress over time results in a reduction in cortisol levels (by first reducing levels of the receptor for cortisol), and this provides a feed-forward mechanism toward the HPA (4.). This feed-forward process results in hypervigilance and anxiety, which are associated with increased inflammation in the body/mind. (See Chapter 4: Protect for more on inflammation and the ECS and the neuroimmune axis.)

The prime role of the ECS in stress has been demonstrated in animals, showing that when the CB1R function is blocked or the receptor level is knocked down, there is an increase in HPA axis activity (adrenocortico-tropic hormone [ACTH] production), both after acute stress and when no stress has been imposed on the animals).[114] The long-term effects of the derangement in cortisol production (along with other glucocorticoids) affects cardiovascular, immune, metabolic, reproductive, and brain health, making us more susceptible to diabetes, heart disease, kidney disease, infertility, mental health problems, and even cancer.[115]

Interoception and the Brain

Both the appealing and the potential adverse effects of THC are associated with our perception of our internal state: hunger, fatigue, sadness, etc. These internal emotional signals are designed to motivate behaviors: "I feel hungry, therefore I will eat." We discussed how this happens with eating and sleeping and the ECS; now, we extend this to feelings of fear and anxiety.

Connectivity in the brain is how brain networks link up during certain activities. These networks consist of anatomical parts of the brain, home to collections of nerve cell bodies. Different types of inputs will increase their interactions or cause them to organize. At a deeper level, these network connections are made by synapses (the space between the cell membranes) where individual neurons transfer information—the neurotransmitters flow across the synapse. The activity in different networks can be measured using a noninvasive tool called functional magnetic resonance imaging (fMRI). fMRI measures blood flow connecting these networks and diagrams the electrical impulses between these different brain regions. The interpretation of the data is a map of the flow of information in the brain: how regions connect and how many parts connect. Some of the things being measured by fMRI are pain processing, attention, how psychedelic drugs affect these networks, and effects of mindfulness meditation.

The insula is a region in the brain thought to be associated with consciousness. It is where we process pain, and is associated with self-awareness, feelings coming from our gut (as in visceral pain or hunger), orgasm, insight, maternal love, and attention to the things that are important or that stand out. Therefore, the insula is thought to be directly associated with interoception. Deficient function of the insula has been associated with autism spectrum behavior, and with the inability to describe emotions (alexithymia). Electrical stimulation of the insula in rats induced pain relief. Mindfulness-based training can change how our perceived bodily sensations help regulate our behavior. This happens through enhancing connectivity between the insula with all of its connecting nodes.[116]

The insula is somewhat of a relay station between three brain networks: the salience network (the area of the brain asking, "Should I pay attention to this?"), the default mode network (DMN—mind wandering when not engaged in a task), and the executive network (used when we need focus, self-control, and problem-solving). The salience network allows for what is coming in through the senses to be routed to the right place for both perception and processing. The DFN, when uncoupled from the other networks, is considered to be our resting mind state; there is not much input from the outside world. But our brains tend to not like this boring state of affairs and seek something either to focus on or distract. It is where we go when we say we have a wandering mind or during creative processes. The wandering mind can be playful and wishful or it can be obsessive, as it is in the situations of anxiety and depression where the self is involved in excessive rumination and introspection. (More on this in Chapter 5: Forget). After childhood trauma, or even adult trauma, the salience network can get stuck, resulting in our mind-wandering state to be focused on the negative, upsetting, scary, sad, or anxious feelings associated with the trauma. This is when we may need outside help from therapy.

Certain therapeutic activities can invoke something called flow state. This is referred to by some as being "in the zone." It is a mental state that we can enter when focused on a single task, without thoughts of self. These activities connect certain regions of the brain to work together more cooperatively. This state has been likened to that of practicing mindfulness.* By entering flow state, it is possible to disconnect the salience network, the

---

* Mindfulness is a mental state that is a practice of focusing on the present moment while at the same time being able to acknowledge feelings, thoughts, or bodily sensations. The aim is to notice the self and not be attached to what is witnessed, but rather acknowledge it and let it pass by.

part of the brain that is interpreting the stimuli coming into the brain. The salience network decides what we should give attention to and predominates in PTSD, depression, and chronic anxiety. Cultivating flow state can help to retrain the brain so that the salience network is no longer prominent, thus helping to relieve depression, anxiety, and traumatic recurring memories (Box 3.3).

BOX 3.3   WHAT IS FLOW STATE?

The opposite of boredom and anxiety.

Strategies for entering flow state:

ALLOW PLENTY OF TIME: Set aside a block of time for the activity where you will have no interruptions. This could be a private space or place where the activity happens. Turn off electronics and plan to not respond to text messages, phone calls, emails, etc. Set a time, at least 25 minutes, and enter the activity completely.

ENTERING A TASK: If what you plan to do is too repetitive or boring it may not induce flow state. The activity needs to be something that is challenging and dynamic for your brain. It can be any activity that provides an experience of complete absorption in an activity.

FOCUS: Focus on your body—take control of your physical capabilities. Focus entirely on the activity, losing self-consciousness.

DOCUMENT: Write about your experience. How did you concentrate? Is your skill increasing? What was the level of challenge for you?

ACTIVITIES: Try surfing, rock climbing, table tennis, swimming, tai chi, trail running, or cycling. Other activities for getting lost in the moment are playing chess or video games, engaging in creative work such as playing music or making art, dancing, cooking/baking.

Some doses of THC have been shown to impair executive function: tasks are harder to complete, and goal-oriented behavior can fall to the wayside. When human subjects were given THC (6 mg) administered by vaporization of cannabis flower, fMRI measurements of their brain showed increased perfusion in the area of the insula. In adolescent cannabis users, activation of the DFN increased compared to non-users (results from a compilation of studies), but also showed increases in the executive function regions.[117] This may be why many cannabis users say that they feel more creative! The mind wanders in a constructive way. Using THC consciously in this way, as a means to problem-solve and promote creativity, could help to bring awareness and increase interoception.

Body/Mind Interface 3

Interoception describes our ability to acknowledge and interpret what is going on in our bodies. Sometimes anxiety or panic are related to feelings in the body, such as the heart rate going up, but a lack of awareness that connects such physical sensations and our emotions can lead to mal-expression of what we feel. Having such unconscious feelings can contribute to challenges of self-regulation. In the form of psychotherapy that was described by Swiss psychiatrist Carl Jung, we all have complexes, or ways of responding/reacting that have been shaped by multiple experiences, events, environments, relationships, and memory images. A commonality across all complexes is that when their energy is activated, they always manifest in the body.

The exercise below is to first bring on, and then move your attention to, uncomfortable body sensations and associated feelings in the body. Second, they are intended to normalize typical body sensations by bringing them to consciousness. Notice any thoughts, feelings, or sensations that are similar to your experience of anxiety or your focus on health worries. Try each one on separate occasions (not one after the other) and self-rate what you would interpret as anxiety on a scale from 0%–100%.

1. Over-breathing: Breathe forcefully, fast, and deep for 1 minute.
2. Hold your breath for 30 seconds.
3. Tense all body muscles for 1 minute.
4. Stare at yourself in a mirror without blinking—2 minutes.
5. Lie down and relax for at least one minute then sit up quickly—1 minute.

If you scored >50%, you may be misinterpreting bodily sensations for anxiety. Other ways that a lack of interoception can manifest include being hungry and expressing it as anger (hangry!), being tired and it being expressed as frustration, and not recognizing emotional signals and becoming distressed or sad.

What Can I Expect to Feel if I Take THC?

The most common experience reported by cannabis users is euphoria. Along with this is a heightened sensory perception (the senses are enhanced) and an altered perception of time (periods of time seem longer than they are). These effects come on quickly when inhaled cannabis is used, but more gradually when consumed orally.

Internally perceived states can also be enhanced by the psychoactive action of THC. The felt effects are likely due to multiple things happening including activation of dopamine neurons, inhibiting the breakdown of acetylcholine and enhancing serotonin release. At higher doses, binding of a serotonin receptor can occur. These things combined have been shown to lead to a decrease in aggressive behaviors (unlike alcohol) as well as reduce feelings of irritability and agitation. Improved social behaviors have also been measured in cannabis users by increasing openness, agreeableness (higher in men), empathy (higher in women), and fairness.[118] Because THC enhances sensory awareness, it can facilitate or increase interoception and may be similar to flow state. Using THC for this purpose works best if you use it in the setting of doing a body/mind activity such as exercise—swimming, yoga, tai chi, surfing, or getting out into nature and taking a slow walk.

Consuming more THC than you intended to, or not understanding what might be too much, can cause a dysphoric experience that presents as acute anxiety, paranoia, acute psychosis, loss of personal identity, and, more rarely, hallucination or delusions (more on this in Chapter 5: Forget). It could be that THC at high dose is over-activating interoception to the point of resembling what occurs in depression, anxiety, schizophrenia, and psychosis—the salience network gets exaggerated. Once you know how you experience THC, you can dial in the dose where you find the smallest dose that provides the most beneficial experience overall.

There is some small evidence that use of CBD along with THC may minimize the psychoactive effects of THC. However, there is also the chance that CBD could inhibit the therapeutic effects of THC (such as pain relief) when taken together. This may depend on the ratio of CBD to THC, but there is no conclusive agreement. It has been suggested that the 1:1 ratio of these two compounds may enhance THC effects (so you don't need as much for the same effect). CBD is considered more socially acceptable due to its different psychoactive profile compared to THC; CBD does not provide the other effects we are mostly talking about in this book. These psychoactive effects are due to the direct activation of cannabinoid receptors by THC. The terpenes don't directly activate cannabinoid receptors but, like CBD, have their own biologic activity.

Stress in our modern lifestyle has broad impacts on our health, including sleep and fertility. Sleep disruption, due to overall AL, is caused by changes in hormone secretions that can contribute to a loss of rhythm in the brain's suprachiasmatic nucleus. The prime hormone that becomes dysregulated is cortisol, which is of utmost importance for modulating our clock gene expression. Further, inadequate sleep increases our response to negative emotional stimulus, which can affect our cardiovascular and endocrine health. Chronic stress can cause elevations of cortisol, or high cortisol in the afternoon, rather than the morning. It can also suppress melatonin, our endogenous hormone made by the pineal gland, which has been associated with infertility. Supplementation of melatonin may be a good adjunctive approach for treating infertility.

Case in Point

My patient is a 46-year-old woman who was coming to see me for her ongoing suffering due to symptoms of long COVID (for more on post-viral syndromes, see Chapter Protect). She experienced a fairly severe form of the illness, recovered, and then had a relapse after drinking some alcohol at a party. She developed chest pain and went to the emergency department 3 times over 5 months. Each time, the doctors performed an EEG and did not find any abnormalities in her cardiac function. Her ongoing symptoms are shortness of breath, decreased endurance for any exercise, dizziness, feeling shaky, brain fog, and low blood pressure. She thinks that she is having heart attacks. She was scheduled for further evaluation by a cardiologist to determine whether she had experienced a cardiac event. This visit resulted in no findings of having had a heart attack. This prompted her to have to re-evaluate the experience she was having as a panic attack.

It is not uncommon, after having any experience where we may have felt betrayed by our body, to develop anxiety around any physical feelings or thoughts that recreate or bring up that betrayal experience. Our threshold for reactivity gets lowered. As an example, it is common for cancer patients to be hypervigilant around any pain they have or other sensations as being a recurrence of cancer.

For the woman I described, who had previously been healthy and never had any health issues, fear had crept in around her health that she was unaware of. She attributed all of her symptoms to a physiologic event. It is highly likely that post-COVID effects were still at play, namely dysfunction in the cells (endothelial) of the blood vessels that were causing some of her symptoms. But it was her reaction to these symptoms that led to panic attacks that she interpreted as heart attacks. Once she was reassured that she was not having heart attack, and she tuned into these feelings as those of anxiety, she was able to address her symptoms using mindfulness and breathwork and greatly improved her quality of life.

If you have ever experienced panic, you may have experienced freezing along with it. Sometimes having to make an everyday decision can release a surge of adrenaline and you are sent backward in time to another event that may have initially triggered your stress response. This type of freezing, or dissociation from present time, is debilitating. A good thing to do in this instance is to curl up into your fetal position and cover yourself with a weighted blanket. Slow your breathing, wrap your arms around yourself, and gently and slowly rock back and forth. This motion is programmed into our brain from the womb and serves to synchronize parts of our brain that enforces relaxing.

If this type of event happens to you and you are with other people, you obviously cannot curl up into a ball and rock yourself! Instead, take a minute to relax your body (learn how to do a progressive relaxation) and then tune into the area of your body where you have the most intense physical sensation. It's fair for you to advocate for yourself in the presence of your friends, state what you need, and let them know what is happening to you. Hopefully you can take a moment to relax into that center, using deep belly breathing, to facilitate body awareness and bring calm. Whenever you feel your center contracting, initiate one of the 2 types of breathing at the end of the chapter. One final approach is to try to match this activated energy with exercise. This can help to drain off the activated energy in the body, in a homeopathic kind of approach (like cures like). You will need to try to find what works best for you.

Women's Health

Women are twice as likely as men to develop any kind of an anxiety disorder. This is likely due to the monthly cyclical changes in estrogen and progesterone or differences in sex steroid between men and women. An imbalance in these hormones, as well as their cyclic fluctuations, can make women susceptible to the development of anxiety. Where a woman is in her reproductive life can also play a role, as the stress response can be exaggerated in peri and postmenopausal women. This may be due to declining levels of estrogen, but could also be associated with too little progesterone. Estrogen also can upregulate dopamine receptors in the brain, and this has been implicated in the setting of postpartum psychosis. Certain genetics and mutations in enzymes that are processing estrogen along with other neurotransmitters (COMT and MAO) can also be involved in estrogen's excitatory effects.

Progesterone is an interesting sex steroid hormone shown to be anxiolytic in itself (as a neurosteroid), as it is considered to be a calming (neuro-inhibitory) compound in the brain. When broken down in the body, the progesterone metabolites allopregnanolone and pregnanolone are also anxiolytic. They have been shown to potentiate the GABA receptor, thereby promoting the slowing of neuronal firing. The amount of progesterone produced at the end of the menstrual cycle, and the ratio of progesterone to estrogen, are partially responsible for premenstrual symptoms and exacerbation of obsessive-compulsive disorder (OCD), and dysphoric disorders (major depressive disorder), especially in postpartum depression (PPD: there is an FDA-approved drug, an analog of allo-pregnenalone, for treating PPD: learn more in Chapter 4: Protect). Premenstrual dysphoric disorder (PMDD) can include irritability, depression, anxiety, or a combination of the 3. Current treatments include OCs, other forms of contraception and antidepressant medications (SSRIs). Another option is focused more on treating the cause using botanical medicines to regulate hormonal function, tackling stress resilience, and treating the HPA axis (again using herbal allies). A multimodal, whole person body/mind approach can provide a world of difference, and in many cases lead to being able to avoid having to be medicated. Some of new research suggests the antidepressants (also used to treat anxiety) have not reduced but have been associated with an actual increase in the incidence of depression. Side effects related to the use of antidepressants can include nausea, weight gain, reduced libido, anorgasmia, and generally feeling flat. Either the current treatments are not working or are having negative consequences. SSRIs are most effective when used in the short term and used when using therapy at the same time.

Let's consider briefly the lived experience of hormonal imbalances is. The up and down of emotions can be debilitating *and* they can also bring self-awareness. Consider that when hormone levels increase, as in during the second half of the menstrual cycle, there can be enhanced brain function due to increase in dopamine activity. When dopamine activity is high, this be experienced as the tendency to have variable and strong emotions. It can also lead to an increase in obsessive-compulsive behaviors, which could be drinking binges or any type of addiction (shopping, overeating, etc.). Some women experience marked anger, increased interpersonal conflicts, insomnia or hypersomnia, feelings of overwhelm, edgy, tense, and overactive mind. Each person can experience some of these things one month and the next month something different. The experiences felt in themselves are not necessarily negative, but the response to the felt experience can significantly disrupt both function and well-being. It can feel like being out of control; sometimes we are! We are under the control of our biochemistry, and we can also alter it.

Consider that if you are having a lot of anxiety, there may be something that needs to be brought to consciousness and be dealt with. The arising of anxiety in itself need not be pathological. It could be the lifting of a veil between the conscious and the subconscious mind. During moon time, we may be more sensitive to the ability to see into ourself, such as unveiling the roles we play and why, examining duties we think we must execute as defined by cultural or societal norms, and seeing more into the mystery of life. The moon time is a gifted time to see behind the veils. We have to trust in our body's wisdom and tune into our intuition. It is a time to feel curious about what is under the veil and work with it rather than suppress it with medications. If you are angry, maybe the feeling is valid and shows you something that needs to be expressed.

It will pay to be in tune with your moon cycle. You can start by simply tracking it on a calendar. The time around ovulation can bring heightened awareness, as well as the week leading up to the moon time. These times can be disruptive or they can be opportunities. We have to learn to work with our biochemistry in the midst of these fluctuations. Veils are a symbol for the sacred too. What is desired is to be able to use the veil at our will, rather than the veil manipulating us. We can employ veils when we don't want anyone to enter our sacred space, as a means up upholding or putting up boundaries. The moon time is a time of descent into our deep places so make space for this in your life. Be alone, engage in psychotherapy, dive into your depths and persist in finding what is spiritual nourishment for yourself.

Of course, if you are having debilitation in the body/mind, seek out help! Having a hormonal map of your cycle can reveal your patterns. Nourishing the adrenal glands can help with reproductive balancing. The thyroid is another piece of the complex endocrine feature for women and you may need help with the function of this gland. We are complex creatures, made for creating life and there is nothing to be ashamed of if you are having problems. The simple act of engaging in social activities and having the social support from other women will provide nurture and strength. Adaptogenic herbs are those that increase our ability to adapt to physical, chemical and biological stressors and are women's herbal allies!

You also need a good healthcare provider who is versed in non-pharmacologic approaches to determine what is the best approach for you. We often cannot make perfect decisions on our own and we can seek help. I suffered with extreme changes that were hormonally induced, resolving completely with menopause. There is no reason to suffer; don't think you can do it on your own or that you must just endure monthly mood swings that can affect quality of life and be debilitating. Get feedback from trusted others and make it a priority to tend to your health.

Another calming hormone is oxytocin, a neurochemical released by the posterior pituitary gland that is an influential player in the neuroendocrine stress response. Getting touched, as in skin-to-skin contact or though massage, can promote the release of oxytocin. Exercise can also stimulate oxytocin release. Oxytocin is the chemical responsible for uterine contractions and for reducing activation of the amygdala in response to fear or anger. Oxytocin has been given intranasally and shown to do this in experimental settings.[119] Oxytocin has also been called the love hormone as it promotes mother/infant bonding after childbirth. Every time a baby suckles the breast, a surge of oxytocin is released to allow for milk to flow. Women across time and over the globe have known the beneficial effects of breastfeeding and the peaceful and relaxing feelings that tend to reduce stress.

Conscious approaches to managing hormonal swings that affect mood include developing a mindfulness practice, practicing deep abdominal breathing, and toning the vagus nerve through this breathing, or—better yet—laughing and singing! Remember the vagus nerve as the wanderer traveling from our brainstem, down the spinal cord where it is the line of communication between our organs and our brain. It regulates our heart rate and breathing. By slowing our breathing, thereby slowing our heart rate, we can calm our nervous system. If you want to know how you are doing in this sympathetic nervous system department, measuring heart rate variability (the interval in between heart contractions) is one of several parameters associated with resilience that is an easy tool to use to gain feedback. This is employed on wearables devices such as Apple watches and others that give you feedback about your health metrics. The lower the variability in your heart rate at rest, a measure of the parasympathetic nervous system (and the vagus nerve), the more stress resilience you have—or a better ability to recover from mental, physical, and emotional stress. Biofeedback training is something that can help you improve your heart rate variability. Breath control influences your physiology by down regulation of inflammation through the vagus nerve, and inflammation exacerbates anxiety.

Vagus nerve stimulators are external devices (they can also be implanted) that send electrical signals to the vagus nerve and have been shown to improve anxiety scores in PTSD and other anxiety disorders. When the vagus nerve is stimulated electrically, it sends signals that facilitate the release of norepinephrine, and can help with the extinction of bad memories, inhibit the sympathetic nervous system, and decrease inflammation. This intervention may be useful in extreme cases, but by engaging the vagus nerve naturally you may find that it brings calm and may also reduce inflammation in the body.

Inflammation is a major player in generating anxiety, so using natural means, such as herbs and phytochemicals, to treat inflammation are important. The microbiome also has a major role in our moods, as microbes are making neurotransmitters. The gut/brain axis is influenced by what we eat, our sleep, medications, infection, and exercise. Eventually we may be able to use microbes as a therapy for mental illnesses. The research has just begun, but we know that a healthy plant-based diet, providing many types of fiber, supports a diversity in the microbiome, and this diversity helps to support mental health.

Using Cannabis for Mood

Cannabis has been understudied as a potential mental health therapy. As stated earlier, the second and third reasons that people who use cannabis for medical reasons say that they use cannabis for anxiety and depression. If you are depressed, then euphoria sounds pretty good, right? The use of cannabis for depression or anxiety can be a double-edged sword however. Cannabis may lift mood or relieve anxiety in the short term, but this is likely a hack and not getting at treating the underlying cause. For the sake of overall well-being and health, the entire body/mind needs attention.

Cannabis use that began in adolescence may *contribute* to the development of anxiety and/or depression as we age. This causation of mental health disruption may depend on the type of use, such as frequency and potency of cannabis used, but overuse and use of high-potency cannabis (such as vape pens, dabbing) will downregulate the ECS and suppress its normal function.

THC can facilitate dopamine release, which could be a good thing in the setting of depression, but not so good for those with bipolar disorder, previous psychosis, or schizophrenia. Depression and anxiety are closely linked; when one is present, often the other is close beside. The complete picture is unclear, but it is known that cannabis use disorder is commonly diagnosed in people who have generalized anxiety disorder (GAD) and major depression. Alcohol use can also exacerbate depression and anxiety. Turning to substances for relief is not uncommon. When comparing alcohol to cannabis, cannabis is less harmful overall. Highly potent cannabis products such as oil, wax, hash, dabs, and vape pens should probably be reserved for occasional use as downregulation ECS function may exacerbate some health issues or mental health conditions.

Cannabis and Pregnancy

Getting pregnant is a concern when using cannabis for PMS or PMDD. Cannabis use during the childbearing years can be tricky, especially if not using birth control. Cannabis use in pregnancy has not been shown to be 100% safe for the developing embryo or fetus. Although it has been shown to be the most commonly used recreational drug by pregnant women (up to 20% report they used cannabis during pregnancy), and this number increased during the COVID pandemic, the relative safety remains under investigation. While not toxic to the developing baby, or known to cause physical birth defects, there is a need to exercise caution with regard to development of the brain and THC.

Because THC loves fat so much, it can easily slide across barriers, such as the blood-brain barrier and the placental barrier. In other words, the placenta keeps the score.[120] THC binds to CBRs both in the placenta and in the developing baby. Research from animal studies describe how important the ECS is in brain development. The ECS machinery is found in the most primordial life forms *and* in the early human central nervous system that is rapidly expanding prenatally, postnatally, and even into our 20s when brain development is complete. Before a woman even knows she has conceived, the ECS has already been at work in the genesis of neurons and other brain cells (glia), migration of neurons, the building of connections in the brain and forming synapses (where neurons communicate), and the pruning of these synapses until young adulthood. Long-term effects of supplementing THC in pregnancy are still not well understood. We know that the CBRs are primary targets of THC, and that they regulate the differentiation of neurons into different types. Prenatal THC exposure results in the CB1R being expressed less often. (It is the most widely expressed protein of its type in the brain!)

The short-term regulation of how our genes is expressed is called epigenetics. Our DNA sequences do not change (this is called a mutation), but nutrients, our emotional/social environment, and exposures to drugs and chemicals can all alter the interpretation of our DNA. Our genes can be turned on or off. Endocannabinoids call out baby neurons and place them into templates in the early brain, along with all of the major neurotransmitter systems: dopaminergic, GABAergic, opioidergic, serotonergic, and glutamatergic. Cannabis use during pregnancy can lead to THC epigenetically turning down the expression of the CB1R during embryonic and fetal development. The loss of CB1R expression affects optimal neurotransmitter systems development. Research suggest that this can affect cognitive function in childhood and adulthood, impact stress resilience, and lead to problems with attention (ADD/attention deficit hyperactivity disorder [ADHD]) and aggressive, defiant, and self-harming behaviors.[121, 122]

The newest information supporting ECS having a homeostatic role in brain development is that even short-term exposures to THC results in rapid changes to the ECS. These changes can affect neurology and psychiatry (neuropsychiatric) phenotypes during development. One risk is for risk for overall substance abuse risk due to changes in the area of the brain associated with reward, driven by dopamine signaling. Research strongly supports that when exposed to cannabis across any of the stages of brain development, there can be individual risks (based on genetics and other environmental factors) that can lead to mental health dysregulation later in life. One study measured increased cortisol and decreased heart rate variability in children whose mothers used cannabis, leading to an increase in anxiety characteristics in childhood and later in life.[123]

> **HERBAN LEGEND #5:** Because cannabis is an herb and our body has an endocannabinoid system it is safe to use in pregnancy. During the current cannabis renaissance, there has been an increasing perception that cannabis use is totally safe, even for pregnancy.

Pregnant women may be looking to alleviate a medical condition, such as nausea and vomiting, management of mood symptoms or to replace alcohol for recreation. The message here is that if you are going to use cannabis during the reproductive years, it is wise to be use birth control or discontinue any cannabis use if you intend to get pregnant. Because of the critical developmental windows occurring early in pregnancy, during the time the embryo is beginning, clean living is in order! No drug in pregnancy is the safest approach for the development of a baby. It remains unclear whether potency or frequency of cannabis use affects the risk. For instance, would drinking a cannabis tea occasionally help with morning sickness vs. smoking a joint every day (more on cannabis and fertility in Protect)? There are more questions than answers.

The risk/benefit ratio of using cannabis at all in pregnancy needs to be weighed by each person. It is known that maternal stress is a significant risk factor for pregnancy outcomes (premature birth, low birth weight) and that maternal stress shapes the developing brain. The effects of stress on development are also epigenetic, influencing development of the nervous system development, the HPA axis, and neurotransmitter signaling. Maternal stress alone affects a baby in development and this can be measured when still in the womb by tracking movement and heart rate changes. Maternal prenatal stress includes depression and anxiety, economic stress, lack of social or family support, catastrophic events, intimate partner violence, and other trauma. Simply having other people with whom to talk, feeling a sense of belonging, and having someone to rely on for practical/material help can reduce the risk of poor pregnancy outcomes.

Anxiety Disorders

Generalized Anxiety Disorder (GAD) affects more than 6 million Americans! First-line therapy is to establish a relationship with a psychotherapist because we can be creating a lot of our anxiety with our mind. Overactivation of the DFN is one link to the over-rumination of negative thoughts that lead to decreased well-being. Learning how to control the active mind and engaging in mindfulness training are imperative.

Antianxiety prescription drugs were first introduced in 1960 with the drug Librium followed by Valium (a benzodiazepine- slows activity in the nervous system by enhancing GABA); they were seen as improvements over the barbiturates (drugs that induce relaxation and drowsiness) that had previous been used. Two decades later it was realized that patients become dependent, addicted, and tolerant to these drugs. In addition, if they are combined with opioid drugs or alcohol they can lead to death by overdose. The most commonly prescribed benzodiazepine drugs are: Valium, Xanax, Ativan and Klonopin. These drugs induce sedation and hypnosis, thereby relieving anxiety, muscle spasms, and seizure. They can however be highly addictive and promote negative effects on health, such as increasing the risk of developing dementia later in life (more on this in Forget), increasing the risk of falls in older adults, suppressing respiration, cognitive impairment, and effects on driving. These risks are particularly relevant for the drugs that have longer-lasting effects (Xanax, Ativan, Klonopin) and when used consistently for more than 3 years.[124]

Prescribing benzodiazepines needs careful consideration by both the doctor and the patient. They can be helpful in the settings of anxiety panic or intractable insomnia and can act quickly, giving people relief from distress. But as the side effects may outweigh the short-term symptomatic benefit, their use should be avoided or at the very least minimized. Deprescribing or tapering off this class of drugs can be challenging; a safely constructed program and medical management is needed to help wean off long-term benzodiazepine use.

Cannabis may be helpful in the setting of GAD, but it is unlikely to cure it by itself. Using cannabis as a low-dose THC supplement to tone the ECS may help with symptoms, but using cannabis along with psychotherapy and other measures (described in the Integrative Health section of this chapter) all need to be on board. Treating the cause (whether trauma-induced, physical health, or mental health) is key; it's usually not just one thing. The body/mind needs attention!

Panic disorder is an acute onset of severe anxiety that comes with a rush in physical and emotional symptoms: racing heat, feeling fain, sweating, nausea, shortness of breath, chills, dizziness ringing in the ears, and others. These attacks can last up to an hour, but most commonly between 5–20 minutes. There can be other physical ailments that could lead to these same feelings in the body, and you may need to see your primary healthcare provider to rule out any medical cause. Most commonly, a doctor will prescribe an SSRI, yet this will likely only be a fix in the short term. Antidepressants are among the most widely prescribed drugs, and their rate has doubled in the past 10 years. There is evidence, however, that use of antidepressants for 10 years or more was associated with a double risk for cardiovascular and coronary heart disease and mortality, and this was primarily in women with an age of about 55–57 years.[125] After 5 years of antidepressant use, there was an increased risk of diabetes compared to those not on antidepressants. Further, a recent review concluded that the serotonin hypothesis—that depression is caused by a serotonin deficiency in the brain—is not well-supported by the scientific literature. Some of the evidence was said to be "consistent with the possibility that long-term antidepressant use reduces serotonin concentration."[126] Women are significantly more likely to develop depression than men and fluctuations in estrogen are closely linked with women's well-being. Estrogen is likely also regulating serotonin levels in the brain.

While anxiety and panic themselves take a huge toll on the human body, it is unclear yet whether the medications typically used to treat these disorders are improving overall health or not. Yoga and cognitive behavioral therapy were found to provide benefits for worry, anxiety, sleep, depressive symptoms, fatigue, and social participation, even 6 months after an intervention combining the 2 therapies. This data highlights the importance of being actively involved in well-being, rather than just relying on medication alone.[127]

Social Anxiety Disorder (SAD): Typically beginning in childhood or adolescence, SAD—the fear of social situations and specifically for being observed when performing, public speaking, or even interacting socially—more commonly affects women than men. This can severely impact quality of life by affecting relationships, work, academic, and social activities. Managing symptoms psychologically, such as using cognitive behavioral therapy (CBT) along with relaxation techniques, exposure techniques, and specific training in conversational and social skills can help to manage symptoms. There are likely genetic factors that predispose people to anxiety disorders, but medical science does not know all of the ins and outs. Neurotransmitters are at play but it is unclear whether current drugs definitively correct any deficiency in these compounds. While in the short term, these pharmaceutical therapeutic agents may be helpful, multimodal approaches are the most effective in the long term.

Separation Anxiety: While separation anxiety most commonly occurs in children, adults can also be insecure and experience separation anxiety. This can occur in adults even when there was no history of a separation anxiety in childhood. This has been found more frequently in patients with depression associated with suicidal thoughts, in people who are socially withdrawn, have extreme sadness, and problems with concentration.

Separation anxiety can occur after the loss of a loved one or by an event such as moving far away from family and friends.

Therapy in a group, family, or as an individual is an essential piece of addressing anxiety disorders. Developing a therapeutic relationship can be healing in itself. There can be physical symptoms associated with all anxiety disorders such as headache, stomachache, dizziness, diarrhea, and chest pain. Left untreated, anxiety can lead to worsening depression, sleep problems, extreme worry, and even OCD. If you think that you have *any* of the symptoms of *any* form of anxiety, it is important to discuss this with your trusted medical healthcare provider. Learning more about the disorder, determining your own individual triggers, managing stress, conversing with others who have a similar experience, and practicing multiple forms of self-care are all important to recover and lead a normal live.

Naturopathic/Integrative/Functional Approaches
Care of the ECS

There are many ways to stimulate your endocannabinoid production. Work on your social connections—strengthen the ones you have or make new ones. Give yourself the gift of massage by a professional or exchange massage with a trusted friend. If you have an intimate partner, practice simply holding one another skin-to-skin without any sexual experience in mind (if you can!). Engaging in moderate exercise (like brisk walks) produces elevations in anandamide, as does laughter (watching comedy) or even fake laughter! Singing, stretching, or any mindful activities such as yoga, tai chi, qigong, mindfulness, breathwork, and singing (vagal toning) are nourishing and toning to your endocannabinoid system. Having a routine of making sure you get emotional/social and biological needs met is survival-promoting. This can be especially true if you had survival challenges when your brain was developing.

Terpene

Linalool is a floral scent found abundantly in species of lavender. Using this as an essential oil can be calming when applied to wrists and temples or diffused into a room. It tends to be a minor terpene in cannabis, but when it is present, the strongly sedative effects are noticeable with dry vaping. Linalool was shown to bind the GABA receptor and help facilitate GABA binding to the receptor (allosteric pharmacology).[ ]

Measuring Allostatic Load

Some of the ways to measure your AL are through serial salivary cortisol, heart rate variability, pulse rate, BMI, C-reactive protein, white blood cell count, blood pressure, serum triglycerides, and HDL.

Herbal Allies

Nerve Tonic Botanicals

Avena sativa's (oat seed) immature grains contain a milk that has been used traditionally for support of the nervous system. It can be used in a tincture or tea.

Passiflora incarnata (passionflower) is good for mental worry and the exhaustion that can come from your brain being too full. It has also been shown to be helpful for anxiety during tapering of benzodiazepine drugs. [128] It has mild sedative effects.[129]

Scutellaria laterifolia (skullcap) is another great herbal ally that is relaxing and mind-calming.[130]

Valeriana officinalis (valerian) is one of the strongest muscle relaxers in the botanical world and may also help promote sleep.[131] (Some of these are covered more fully in Chapter 2: Sleep.)

Lavendula angustifolia (lavender) is an aromatic plant that originated in the Mediterranean; there are many species. The essential oil component has long been considered to be calming with the ingredient linalool, which is known to bind to GABA receptors. Drinking this as a tea, using as a tincture, or using the essential oil in a hot bath when you are energetically aroused can help with relaxation.

Nepeta cataria (catnip) is a member of the mint family that grows wild all over the world and is known as an attractant for cats. Smelling nepetalactone induces cats to want to rub all over the plant. This plant has been used as a calming agent for body and mind, and may also soothe the gastrointestinal tract.

Hypericum perfatorum (**St. John's wort**) is native to Europe and was considered a holy herb during the Middle Ages. It is sometimes used in the treatment of depression, but this should be managed under the care of someone knowledgeable about the plant. It has been studied for social anxiety disorder and as an antidepressant. It may lead to increased serotonin levels, so should not be used alongside other antidepressants that affect serotonin levels. It can also cause photosensitivity, leading to sunburn. It's great as a topical for wound healing, too.

Humulus lupulus (**hops**), is most commonly associated with alcohol preparation (beer), and has been used for antibacterial properties (why it was originally added to beer) to promote sleep and to treat anxiety and sleeplessness. This plant was originally the only other plant in the same family of cannabis (*Cannabaceae*). The strobile is the flower-like part of the plant that produces a resin full of phytochemicals that have various actions. The volatile oil of the plant is considered to be sedative, while xanthohumol may be cancer-protective; 8-prenylnaringenin has the highest estrogenic activity of any plant.[132] This makes for a great herbal ally during menopause.

Corydailis yanhusuo is a mild sedative and tranquilizing herb that has been used across Asia, also as a pain reliever. By relieving pain and relaxing tissues it can ease anxiety. It is in the same plant family as poppy, but the active ingredient is not an opioid. Corydalis is *not* for use in pregnancy and you should consult with a knowledgeable person prior to using this; there can be toxicity issues.

Adrenal Tonic Herbs/Adaptogens

Glycyrrhiza glabra (**licorice**), is a sweet root—a plant grown and native to Eastern Europe, the Middle East, and Asia. It has long been used to support adrenal function and contains a compound that helps to keep cortisol in circulation for longer periods of time (by inhibiting the enzyme that inactivates cortisol).[133] This is a trusted and safe herb, but caution is advised if you have high blood pressure as glycyrrhizin may reduce potassium levels and has been reported to lead to irregular heart rhythms. This is a great natural sweetener and is also a liver protectant. A cup of licorice tea is soothing to the entire digestive tract. It is a great addition to herbal mixtures as it has properties to help phytochemicals move into tissues and cells.

Withania somnifera (**ashwaganda**), is a small shrub that is native to the Middle East, India, Western China and belongs to the nightshade family (along with tomato, potato, pepper, goji berry). It is a traditional Ayurvedic medicine, known in the herbal world as an adaptogen. The name literally translates to dream carrier (somnifera). Adaptogens in general are intended to help us cope with stress. It is known for toning the adrenal glands and immune system as well as helping with sex steroid hormone balance in both women and men. It may also be acting on GABA and this along with the other properties make it ideal for addressing stress and promoting resilience. This plant is also known as Indian ginseng. I like using it in a tincture in combination with licorice and Chinese or American ginseng. Any product used should be standardized for the active ingredients, withanolides, a group of compounds responsible for the adaptogenic ability. Ashwaganda can help to normalize cortisol, lower pulse rate and blood pressure.

Urtica diocia (**stinging nettle**) is a common unwanted plant growing as a weed that causes stinging to the skin when touched. It is considered a tonic herb and also eaten as a nourishing food when first emerging in the spring, high in iron and micronutrients. Good for strengthening and toning the whole of systems, stinging nettle can be great for addressing fatigue or weakness associated with anxiety or depression. This is one plant ally that is completely safe for pregnancy and lactation and may even help with milk production.

Panax quinquefolius (**American ginseng**) can help for recovery after panic fright or extreme stress and supports immune function. This is another valuable adaptogenic plant, not related to Siberian ginseng (eleuthero) or Korean ginseng (panax). It can help with normalizing glucose levels, increasing the ability to focus, and is thought to be more relaxing than the Asian ginsengs that are stimulating. The medicine is made from the root of the plant

Hormone Balancing Herbs or Hormonal Adaptogens

Angelica archangelica (**Dong qui**) supports estrogen and is more specific for menstrual irregularities rather than PMS. It can be helpful for pelvic pain from fibroids or pelvic congestion by helping with circulation. It can potentially exacerbate hot flashes.

Vitex agnus castus (**chasteberry**) contains chemicals that can help with PMS as a natural way to balance estrogen and progesterone. It does not contain hormones, but acts on the pituitary gland. It can be effective at low dose of up to 50 mg taken in a tincture 2–3 times per day. It is indicated for menstrual cramps, PMS, menstrual migraines, and breast tenderness.[134]

Humulus lupulus (**hops**) contains the strongest phytoestrogen: 8-prenylnaringenin (8PN). 8PN has been shown to have the highest binding affinity to estrogen receptor of any phytochemical tested.

Trifolium praetense (**red clover**) Evidence for the phytoestrogenic activity of *Trifolium* species in grazing animals first revealed that clover isoflavones are weak estrogenic molecules (also found in *Glycine max*, or soy) and some *Fabaceae* family members. Red clover and soy share similar but distinct chemical profiles; both contain genistein, daidzein, formononetin, and biochanin A. Considered to be safe to use in pregnancy as nutritive to the uterus, but may not be recommended for use in situations of estrogen dominance including breast cancer and uterine cancer.

Aromatherapy

Salvias (**sage**), **lemon**, *Ylang ylang*, and **lavender** are not recommended to ingest as essential oils as they can be sensitizing over time (activating the immune response, like an allergy) and also toxic to the liver, kidney, or brain.

Avoid stressful situations. Learn to say no! Stress is caused by unmet expectations and feeling overwhelmed by the amount of emotional input that puts us over the edge of our management abilities. Prioritizing leisure time is an integral piece for regaining control of your HPA and relieving your daily pressure. I have a routine of moving out of my work space and into my back yard daily for some sun and stretching on the grass. My partner and I typically turn on music that we like and lie in our reclining lawn chairs and simply take in the sky and the birds and whatever else enters our consciousness. We may have adapted in our life to constantly perform and this manifests as overwork, an inability to relax, and the desire to be perfect in exchange for thinking we will get the fulfillment we seek. But inner fulfillment will never come from things we do outwardly. Work on letting everything go and perfecting laziness! Make extending kindness to yourself a daily practice and take care of the relationships you value.

Here are 2 methods of breathing to try if you find yourself in a stress-inducing moment.

1. Pursed lip breathing

This one is simple and easy, but extremely effective. The general idea is to breathe out for double the amount of time of your inhalation. Pursed lip breathing helps release air that's trapped in the lungs, and decreases the number of breaths you take while extending exhalation.

Sitting up as straight as you can with relaxed shoulders, take a normal breath for about 4 counts. Then pucker your lips up (think of your mouth when you're about to whistle—that's what your lips should look like) and exhale for 8 counts.

2. Diaphragmatic breathing

Also known as belly or abdominal breathing, this is the granddaddy of breathing exercises, as you're training the body to let your diaphragm do all the work. Your goal here is to breathe through your nose and focus on how your belly fills up with air.

You can do this one either sitting up very straight or lying down. With your shoulders back, keep one hand on your chest and the other on your belly. As you breathe in deeply for about 4–6 seconds, your belly should stick out a bit. Feel the air expanding your stomach and then breathe out slowly, feeling your stomach contract, for a count of 8–12 seconds using the pursed lips as in the first exercise. I find it's nice to do while in bed to help wind down.

Food/Nutrition: Eat an anti-inflammatory diet. The Whole 30 plan is a good fit for this. Stay away from highly processed foods and simple sugars (sweets, candy, desserts). Flood your diet with color; eat a rainbow every day. Guineensine is a compound found in black pepper and long pepper that may help keep your AEA hanging around longer, so spice up your food![135]

Supplements

Lithium orotate is one of my favorites for edginess—up to 20 mg twice per day.

Magnesium threonate is what I turn to for calming the brain, great either before bedtime or in the morning for improved focus—or both.

The B vitamins, taken in a complex, support central nervous system health (B12 is specific) and neurotransmitter synthesis. B12 is best used sublingually. B6 is especially important if you use oral contraceptives.

L-theanine is a compound found in green tea also shown to reduce salivary cortisol and may have a calming effect for some.

Methylfolate is important to support the methylation cycle and epigenetic processes. There are 2 common gene mutations in the general population in an enzyme that converts dietary folate (from foliage) to its usable form. Make sure your vitamin has methylfolate, not folic acid.

Yoga/Chakra

The second chakra, *svadhisthana* means one's abode. The color orange is associated with this chakra. This chakra is most closely associated anatomically with our adrenal glands and the area over the sacrum. It is associated with creativity, aesthetics, procreation, emotions and the unconscious. It is related to the element of water. Sound baths and hot soaking in water will stimulate this chakra. It governs our joy and enthusiasm. By engaging with this chakra, we can find balance, stop seeing things as black and white, and stream our personal choices in life. Cat/cow or extension and flexion of the spine, lunges, and spinal twists such as parivrtta sukhasana and utkatasana konasana, the goddess pose while strongly engaging your core is empowering. With each breath, deepen your squat.

Consider inverted yoga poses as they may help to increase blood circulation to the brain, help regulate neurotransmitters, and nourish the HPA axis.

Balasana: Also known as child's pose, this posture is calming and relaxing and resembles the fetal position. Sit on your heels, then lower your hips to your heels and try to place your forehead to the floor. Place your knees together, if comfortable, or have your knees spread apart—however you can situate so that you can bring your forehead down to the floor. Place your arms alongside your body, with your hands near your feet and palms facing the sky. If needed, you can use any kind of prop to make you more comfortable. You need to adjust to find what works best for you to be able to completely relax in this position.

As a restorative and calming posture, you want to be comfortable so that you can breathe slowly and gently. Relax your belly completely so that your abdomen presses against your thighs on the inhale. Breathe in a slow deep belly breath and hold for 4 seconds and slowly exhale for 8 seconds. Do this for up to 12 breaths. To release, place the palm of your hands just under your shoulders and slowly roll your spine up into your seated position.

Uttanasana: For this standing forward bend, begin in a standing position with feet hip-width apart, inhale, and then slowly exhale and begin hinging at the hips. You want to keep the knees slightly bent and the back flat. You are pulling the head down so that the crown of your head is reaching for the ground and your spine is going to stretch. Breathe deeply as with child's pose and try to stay relaxing into the position for up to 12 breaths. To sum up, bend the knees and roll the spine until you are fully standing again.

Kirtan is a great way to bring in the breathwork, a call-and-response chanting practice of Bhakti yoga: Krishna Das, Jai Uttal, Snatam Kaur, Wynne Paris, and Sita Devi are vocalists you can join with. The more relaxed your throat is, the deeper the note you will be singing. Let it vibrate in your chest as you practice this in a setting where you are either alone or you don't care if someone hears you. This activates the vagus nerve to produce a calming effect.

Developing Physical Courage as a Practice

Physical courage is how you participate in the world—whether you feel brave, strong, resilient, or aware of your limitations. Keeping the body healthy, strong, and resilient is a way to prepare yourself for any type of challenge, not just physical types. Examples of physical courage include activities such as surfing, skydiving, or any physical event, including the training for the event. It requires a certain type of courage to visit a doctor or try new experiences. A lack of physical courage is highlighted by avoiding anything you perceive as a challenge or anything that is a new experience. Developing physical courage requires self-discipline, goal-setting, sometimes working up a sweat, or doing something you have been afraid of—that you think is difficult or dangerous. As you build your resilience to stress, you will naturally build physical courage.

When you engage the executive network by doing these activities, you enter what is called the flow state. (More about this in Chapter Forget.)

Trials of Cannabis for Interoception Enhancement
Enter the time, type, and potency of product and the effects you experience.

Trials	Date/ Time	Oral/ Inhaled	Dose/ Product	Body Awareness	Mind Wandering/ Creativity	1 Hour	2 Hours	3 Hours
1								
2								
3								
4								

Trials of Cannabis for Anxiety

Enter the time, type, and potency of product and the effects you experience.

Trials	Date/ Time	Oral/ Inhaled	Dose/ Product	Anxiety Score Before	Anxiety Score After: 1 Hour	Anxiety Score After: 2 Hours	Anxiety Score After: 3 Hours
1							
2							
3							
4							

Protect

Overview

It was long thought that the brain was an entirely separate organ from the rest of the body: untouched ,and protected from what happened outside the brain. It had a certain privilege. Privilege was supposed to be insured by a border wall, the brain's supposed uncrossable line called the blood-brain barrier (BBB). It is now known that there is a unique network of the tiny blood vessels (microvasculature) in place to heavily *restrict* movement of things in the blood and lymph systems across the BBB, and this is critical for healthy brain function. However, the BBB can break down in the settings of infection, inflammation, and disease.

The vascular and lymph systems are allowing for communication between the brain (or central nervous system) and the rest of the body (periphery). A prime role for the BBB is to protect the brain from infection, toxic compounds produced by bacteria, fungus, and viruses (exotoxins), disease, and to keep it free from inflammation by preventing immune cells from migrating into the brain where they can cause inflammatory damage to nerves. There are scenarios in which the brain calls on immune cells to help with damage control, or clean up after damage in the brain which can occur with traumatic brain injury (TBI), radiation, or any time neural cells are damaged. The ECS influences a variety of dysregulations that can result in poor memory function, changes in appetite, mood, pain, and immune activation.[136]

This fragile ecosystem of the BBB is made of tight connections between the cells that line the BBB (i.e., endothelial cells (ECs)) a construction similar to that of the tight junctions in the gut barrier (discussed in Chapter Eat). The difference between the two barriers is that the tiny blood vessels that run up behind the ECs (i.e., microvasculature) in the BBB have no pores, unlike those intestinal epithelial cells lining the gut. This provides a reduced chance of any leakage. This layer of ECs backs up to the choroid plexus in the ventricles of the brain, the compartment where cerebrospinal fluid (CSF) is made.

All of this description is intended to illustrate the critical importance of protecting our body's electrical and operating systems (the central nervous system: the brain). The job at the BBB is to tightly regulate what goes in and what comes out; the body is an ecosystem in a delicate balance. The term immunoception, or bidirectional monitoring and control of brain-regulated immunity, has been used to describe how the brain is continually sensing and helping to regulate what is happening in the body.[137] This suggests that not only is communication occurring between the body/mind, but that the brain can help to induce the most appropriate immune response to restore homeostasis. Not surprisingly, the endocannabinoid system (ECS) is a primary means of transmitting immune information from the brain to the periphery and vice versa.

Loss of BBB function is found in neurological diseases: multiple sclerosis, stroke, brain tumors, epilepsy), post-viral syndromes, stroke, TBI, and damage from cancer radiation therapy. Just outside the microvasculature of the BBB, there is a basement membrane, a layer of smooth muscle cells, and the CB1R is found on both the ECs and the smooth muscle. The role of the CB1R on these sites is related to the blood vessel ability to dilate and contract but also to limit activation by inflammatory agents.

Nerve cells, called glia, park themselves just next to the border wall (BBB). Glia used to be thought to have a minor role as supporting cells but now we appreciate these glia as very active players in the nervous system. Glia include astrocyte cells, Schwann cells (for neuronal insulation), and microglia (immune cells that are residents in the brain) all of which are involved in nutrient and waste transport between nerve cells. They perform services to support the neurons, each neuron having at least 10 glia servants. The glial cells also have cannabinoid receptors (CB1R and CB2R) that function in the relaying of information both between neurons and from outside the brain.[138] The ECS is involved in BBB homeostasis, contributing by carrying danger messages into the brain and by modulating the brain's inflammatory response to infection. The ECS is a system that transcends tissue barriers and plays a starring role in the communication across tissues, particularly when relaying news about immune responses in the body.

The nervous system is no longer thought to be immune privileged, or isolated by the BBB as evidenced by the field of neuroimmunology. Immune molecules* are considered to be important contributors to our behavior, our brain development, and how our neuronal circuits function. This means that there is a lot more crosstalk going on between the immune and nervous systems than was ever thought before. It is imperative to gain more understanding of this particularly with the relevance to neurological diseases and emerging post-viral syndromes such as long COVID. This is yet another piece of our body/mind wholeness.

Synopsis of Immunity

There are 2 main ways that our immune system functions: offensive mode (innate) and defensive mode (adaptive). The offense is the initial response to an intruder and the defense keeps the intruder out in the future. The basic goal of immune function is to eliminate anything that is "not me." The innate immune response is the one that we are born with, or inborn (natural, gene-coded) set of reactions, intended to protect us from harmful proteins or pathogens (virus, bacteria, fungus parasites, or other microorganisms that can cause disease) that can enter our body. This is the first line of defense in the immune response, sort of like first responders at an accident or the Marines in a military escalation. The cells participating in the innate response are a huge arsenal of warriors that work in cooperation

---

* Immune molecules include antibodies, cytokines, chemokines, interferons, interleukins, stimulating and growth factors.

with each other. This includes neutrophils, mast cells, platelets, B-cells, T-cells, macrophages, all equipped with ECS machinery.

An example of how the innate immune response works is to look at a virus, such as COVID or the flu that crosses the airway/lung barrier, called the mucosa; we become the host to an unwelcome guest. There are genetically-encoded protein receptors called pattern recognition receptors (PRP) programmed to recognize repeating patterns found on pathogens, known as antigens. These antigen codes are called pathogen-associated molecular patterns (PAMPs). As soon as a PAMP is detected, an immediate pro-inflammatory cascade begins, and this entire team activates the inflammasome: a molecular factory for the inducible inflammatory response. Among the first responders getting involved in this process are neutrophils and macrophages. These cells lie in wait, patrol the body, and then put the rest of the immune team on alert by sending out the initial signals. Because of being the sensors and the beacons, they are known as antigen-presenting cells (APCs—platelets, macrophages, dendritic cells, and B-cells). These signals travel to the brain by a wave of information that flows through the blood, lymph, and into the nervous system. The brain's reaction to signaling that an invader is on the premises include inducing fever, reducing appetite, and conserving energy. The brain also plays a role in activating the immune system further by signaling through the vagus nerve to the spleen, which is like a warehouse for immune-related stuff (cells, antibodies). This is the hypothalamic-brainstem-spleen axis (HBS axis), an integral piece of the negative feedback loop for neuro- and systemic immunity, known as the neuroimmune reflex, discussed later.

An Analogy

I took up surfing about 12 years ago. There is certain surf etiquette, which not everyone follows, that is intended to keep everyone safe. I am on my surfboard, paddling as fast as I can, to catch the wave coming up behind me. I love to close my eyes to detect the feeling of the wave propelling my board forward, signaling to me that I have caught the wave (or that it has caught me!). Once I feel this, I open my eyes and surveil to the right and left of me to make sure that I am not going to take off into the path of another surfer. If I see someone already standing on their board riding the wave, particularly if we are going the same direction (either right or left on the wave), then it is my responsibility to pull off the wave in favor of the person who stood up first and is already riding the wave.

On a particular day in which waves were hard to catch, I felt the pull of the wave. Seeing no one to my right or left, I popped onto my board and moved down the line going left on the curl of the surf. Unfortunately, another surfer also decided to pop up on this wave and did not look for me prior to making his move. Although he was to my left, he took off going to the right; we were on a collision course. What the other surfer did is called dropping in and considered not to be good etiquette. In this case, I have the right-of-way and understanding this is of prime importance (many beginning surfers don't know this). What does this have to do with immunity?

The analogy is that I am representing the host and the other surfer is like a pathogen dropping in. He either has to pull off the wave or we collide. Pulling off the wave is what we want the pathogen to do. It is likely that I am going to have an innate reaction to yell at him to get him to pull off the wave! This is what the innate immune response is. The ECS is part of a 'shout out' to the invader. It is non-specific, so any kind of surfer on any kind of surfboard might get shouted at (any kind of pathogen).

The Immune Cascade

The immune system has a chain of command, starting with signals in the blood known as the cytokine response, the beginning of a cascade of events. (See Figure 4.1.) These cytokines then signal to different types of white blood cells, the immune cells (macrophages, mast cells, neutrophils, etc.). The figure depicts a macrophage cell binding an antigen (pathogen or invader) through the PRP receptor and the resulting release of cytokines and reactive oxygen species* (ROS).

---

* ROS are highly reactive chemicals derived from oxygen: peroxides, superoxide, hydroxyl radical. We need antioxidants to quell these reactions and reduce tissue injury that comes from oxidative damage.

FIGURE 4.1   IMMUNE SYSTEM'S CHANGE OF COMMAND

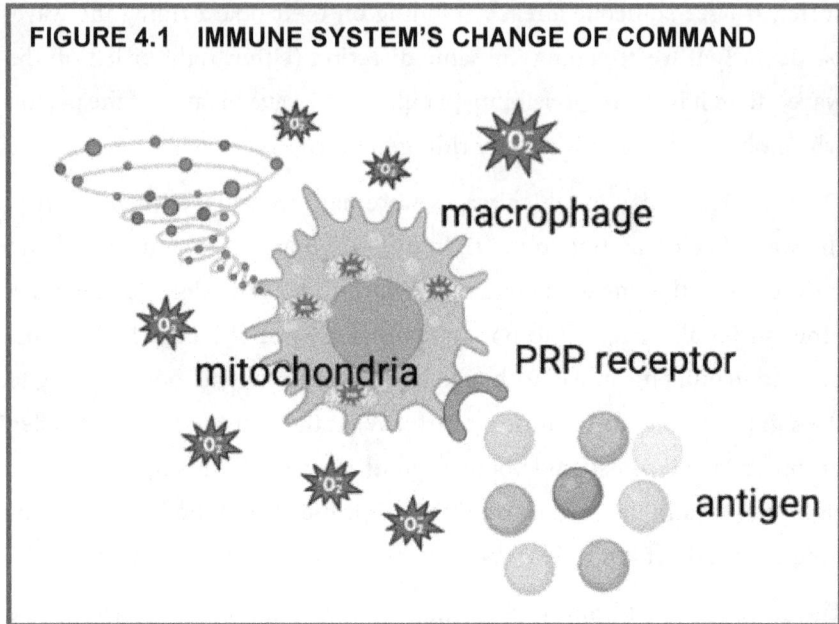

The macrophage, acting as an antigen-presenting cell, prepares to present the antigen to other immune cells so that they can join the battle. The macrophage is already starting to produce cytokines (see the cytokine storm?) and ROS (like hydrogen peroxide and nitric oxide). This takes a lot of energy on the part of the cell, needing to upregulate its energy source, the mitochondria. The mitochondria also produce neurosteroids (made from cholesterol—the human brain weighs 2% of the body's total weight but contains 25% of the cholesterol in the human body) to protect the brain from inflammation.

One of these compounds, pregnenolone, once thought to be a biologically inactive steroid, has been shown to modulate CBRs, which are found on mitochondria.* THC has been shown to increase the level of pregnenolone, an approach for addressing neuroinflammation in the brain. In turn, pregnenolone has been shown to selectively reduce CB1R activity at a subcellular pathway when activation of CB1R has been excessive (JAK-Stat pathway).[139]

---

* A compound that 'modulates' a protein receptor may not directly activate the receptor, but it may help either to facilitate activation or to inhibit activation.

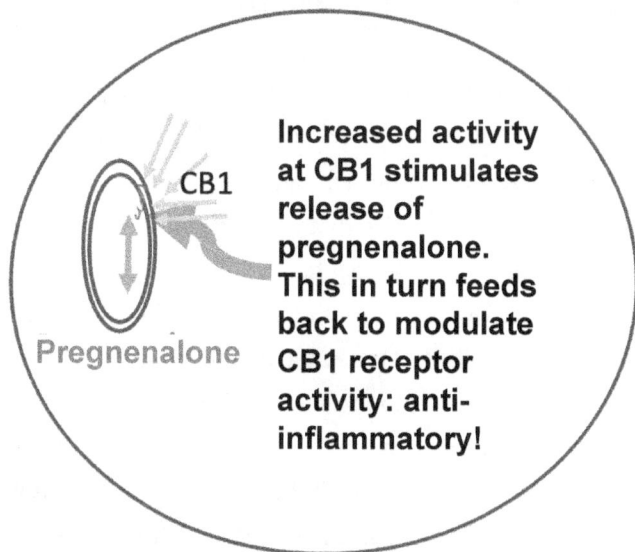

FIGURE 4.2   PREGNENALONE AND CB1R FEEDBACK

CB1

Increased activity at CB1 stimulates release of pregnenalone. This in turn feeds back to modulate CB1 receptor activity: anti-inflammatory!

Pregnenalone

This is an ECS negative feedback loop depicted in Figure 4.2. The CB1R also acts at the mitochondria to squelch the ROS being produced by both infection and the increased cellular activity. You can see how the ECS is thus involved in the immune response at a basic subcellular level and in an ancient cellular inclusion.

The immune response also includes release of endocannabinoids. Endocannabinoids are involved in regulating host defense in a number of ways: activating neutrophils, directing immune cells to move into tissues (migration), directing immune cells to clean up damage (phagocytosis), and serving as a storage unit for making other lipid signalers (such as leukotrienes). Perhaps the best way to describe this is that the ECS provides negative feedback for the whole immune concert through the CB receptors expressed on immune cells. Platelets and APCs, which patrol the lining of blood vessels and tissues, when activated release endocannabinoids, which can act as chemical attractants to call in other immune cells. Contrarily, they are also there also to limit the immune reaction in a yin-and-yang-style relationship with immunocompetence.

The immune defensive team's adaptive immunity is the second-line immune response and includes the programming of T- and B-cells—this supports a finely tuned approach toward specific invaders. The fine-tuning or programming of immune cells ensures that these defensive cells are primed should the same invader come knocking again. When the immune system has adapted in this way, it is like our endogenous vaccination since we develop proteins known as antibodies that are sent out to trap the invaders and render them ineffective. Now adapted, when the cells are alerted that the same invader has returned, there is a swift and efficient response that does not require as much effort as the initial innate response. These cells, as with all immune cells (and red blood cells), are born in the marrow of our bones. The number of cells involved increases in number rapidly when an APC alerts them, by pulling them out of lymph tissue (such as lymph nodes and spleen) into the bloodstream along with stimulating bone marrow to make more cells.

The ECS Provides That We Are Protected

When I studied immunology in medical school, we learned all of the fine detail of these immune cascades. We also learned about chronic inflammation and how it affects the body. What we did not learn: What in the body is supposed to resolve inflammation and prevent or fend off chronic inflammation? What provides for immune system homeostasis? There has to be a negative feedback loop to let the immune response know that the job is done and that the immune cells can all go home. Otherwise, chronic and unchecked inflammation is the result. (Home is the lymph tissues, glands, patches, and the spleen). Turns out that there is a negative feedback system in the immune system and again it is the ECS.

AEA (or anandamide, the bliss molecule) plays a role in daily homeostasis of immune responses, including neuroprotection. It can inhibit some cytokines and also the release of nitric oxide as well as inhibit migration of neutrophils. With a sudden onset of inflammation, 2AG will be upregulated as will the CB2R, with an infection or also in the setting of chronic inflammation (like with an autoimmune disease such as multiple sclerosis).

2AG binding the CB2R activates pathways that modulate the immune response, most notably by turning down the volume on immune mediators or shifting the immune system toward repair (homeostasis). This has been well demonstrated in animal models of multiple sclerosis, hepatitis, hepatitis, stroke injury, lung inflammation, and sepsis (infection in the blood rather than in a tissue). When cannabinoid receptors are knocked down in mice, they have a more severe inflammatory phenotype.[140]

Cannabis (or phytocannabinoids, primarily THC) is well established as having immune modulating potential. Our endocannabinoids (ECBs) modulate immunity, which is a different process than suppressing the immune system. Immune cells will express both CB1R and CB2R. It is not thought, nor has it been demonstrated in humans, that using cannabis can prevent the innate or adaptive immune response from occurring. This has, however, been implicated in some animal studies. Studies using immune cells have shown us that the CB2R is involved in the migration of immune cells and in turning down the volume on inflammatory compounds, such as inhibiting cytokine production.[141, 142] CB1R is also a mediator of immune modulation and is expressed as a normal component of the immune cell. This indicates that the gene for expressing this receptor is always turned on in what is known as constitutive activity.

CNR2 is the gene encoding CB2R, and the expression of this gene is upregulated in the process of inflammation—leading to more CB2R. Monocytes from cannabis users vs. non-users have been shown to have a reduced ability to migrate, and this is likely due to the down regulation of the CB1R on these cells.[143] This can be a positive thing, particularly in the setting of neuroinflammation, where a prime strategy of drug therapies is to keep immune cells out of the brain. One interesting thing about the CB2R is that it does not appear to be found in the human brain when there is no active inflammation. Its expression will be upregulated upon initiation of inflammation and it will be co-expressed with CB1R on glial cells (specifically microglia—the resident macrophage of the brain) and also on immune cells that migrate into the brain due to the breakdown of the BBB.

Neuroimmune Axis

The HBS axis also involves some of the same neurons that activate the adrenal glands (corticotropin hormone-releasing neurons). This is an ancient evolutionary machinery for the neuroimmune axis, illustrating how the brain shapes immunity, beginning with neurotransmitters. Immune cells have receptors for neurotransmitters, explaining in part how this communication occurs—the ECS is a piece of this transmission. Both the immune system and the brain were originally thought to be autonomous. Today we know that the two work in concert for survival and adaptation to stress and threat—not in isolation.

FIGURE 4.3   VAGUS NERVE SIGNALING

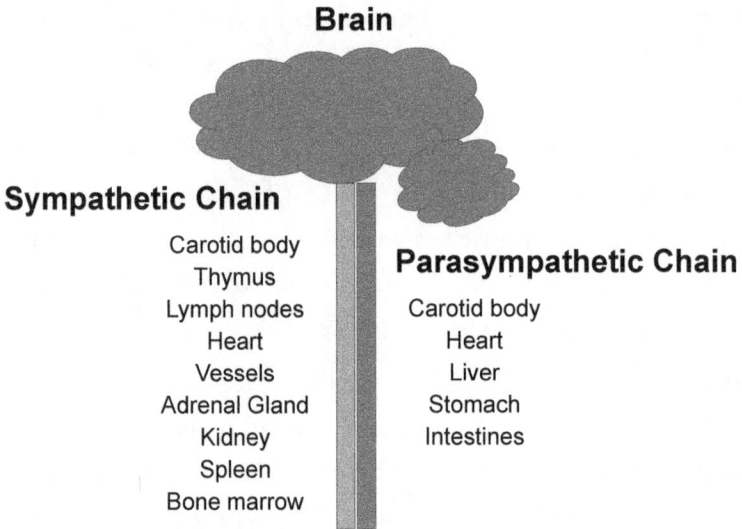

Brain

Sympathetic Chain

Carotid body
Thymus
Lymph nodes
Heart
Vessels
Adrenal Gland
Kidney
Spleen
Bone marrow

Parasympathetic Chain

Carotid body
Heart
Liver
Stomach
Intestines

There is a part of the hypothalamus near the brain's CSF reservoir (ventricles); it is well placed as an immune sensory area. This is where immune cells and other mediators cross the BBB. The CSF is like a quasi-lymphatic system (see the next section for information on glymphatics). When we get an infection, such as a virus that affects our lungs (like the flu or COVID-19), cytokines and other tissue metabolites are involved in weakening the BBB and gaining passage into the brain and which neurons have receptors for. Anytime we are sick, the brain and normal nerve activity is altered. This can be illustrated by the onset of fever, how we lose appetite, feel tired, and can have brain fog when we start getting sick—we need this prompt response telling us to slow down.

When the cytokine signals are received by the brain, which can also occur through signaling *up* the vagus nerve *to* the brain. As soon as the signal is received, there is activation of the vagus nerve going *away* from the brain and back *down* to the spleen through the splenic nerve and to other organs (Figure 4.3).[144] We also need this immediate response as a protective measure, as infection is an acute stressor on the body. The spleen monitors constantly for blood-borne organisms and antigens. The spleen is in touch with the brain via the sympathetic chain, which is signaling with noradrenaline and then acetylcholine. This communication occurs because T-cells and B-cells are housed in the spleen (along with other cells) and so they are sent into the bloodstream and into tissues to do their jobs (similar to calling the fire department).

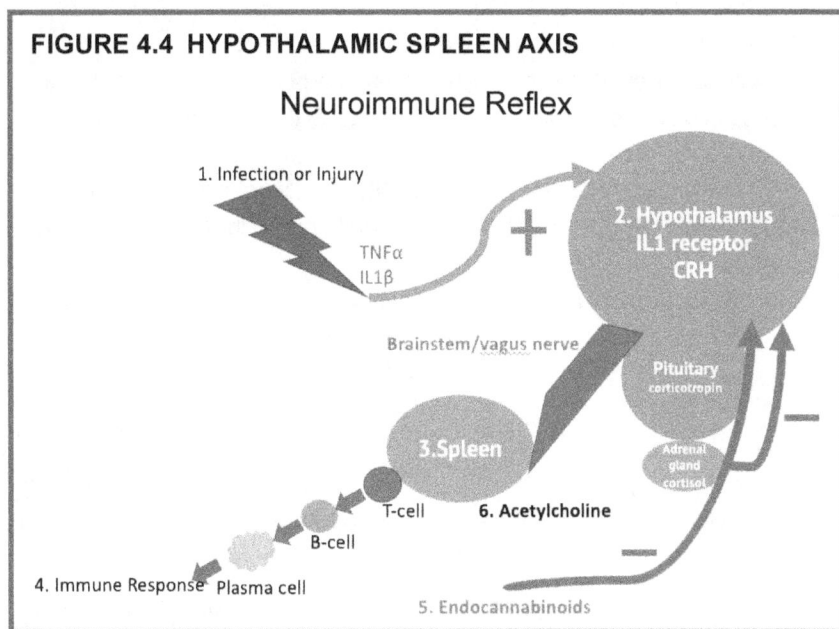

FIGURE 4.4 HYPOTHALAMIC SPLEEN AXIS

Neuroimmune Reflex

1. Infection or Injury

TNFα
IL1β

2. Hypothalamus
IL1 receptor
CRH

Brainstem/vagus nerve

Pituitary
corticotropin

3.Spleen

Adrenal
gland
cortisol

T-cell   6. Acetylcholine

B-cell

4. Immune Response Plasma cell

5. Endocannabinoids

Once inflammation and the immune response has been called into action and is doing its job, then there needs to be resolution of the inflammation. This is where the HSA axis comes into play (Figure 4.4; see Box 4.1

for description). The upregulation of endocannabinoids has a role in this, through activation of CB2R. The influx of endocannabinoids works deactivating immune cell migration and cytokine production in an effort to bring the system back to homeostasis. Macrophage (or monocyte) cells are central for both the interface between the body/brain and also for resolution through the HSB reflex. The activation and smooth operation of the ECS is central to this process, and specifically the CB2R is an important target for resolving the immune response and dampening pro-inflammatory mechanisms. This is because by modulating release of TNFa, IL6, and IL1b will stop the cascade.

BOX 4.1   THE NEUROIMMUNE AXIS

1. Infection or tissue injury starts the cascade.
2. This triggers the sending of signals to the brain where the IL1b receptor activates the vagus nerve.
3. The vagus nerve release of norepinephrine triggers more of the immune cells into action.
4. The innate and adaptive response are happening.
5. Endocannabinoids along with cortisol, produced by the HPA axis (this is a stress on the body) signal back to the brain to help resolve inflammation.
6. The vagus nerve signals again to the spleen where acetylcholine is released for calling the immune cells home, back to the lymph tissues.

Glymphatics

A recent discovery around 2013-15 has further changed how we view the immune privilege of the brain.[145] A system in the CNS for clearing waste from the brain, made of channels akin to the lymph system in the periphery, was imaged and described. A lymph network travels alongside our blood vessels draining fluid from the tissues to circulation, to help balance our body fluids, and also carries immune cells to their destinations (it's like our body's sewage system). The glymphatic system has been found to turned on by sleep. In this case, the glymphatics are important for delivering cholesterol and other lipids to the brain (remember pregnenolone?), maintaining fluid homeostasis in the brain by draining excess fluid (too much fluid in TBI and in neurologic diseases), and helps to clear cytokines from the brain. Impaired function of this drainage system is a component of neuroinflammation.[146]

Most of this takes place when we are asleep. You can see the importance of good flow, draining the brain, and calming inflammation for optimal health. Cannabinoids can also help heal and close the BBB to ensure that the brain is not impaired or compromised by ongoing inflammation.

In a study of people with HIV (pHIV), where the inflammation from the virus and the virus itself crosses over into the brain, neuroinflammation does not resolve on its own—even with current therapies—to treat the HIV infection (antiretroviral therapy). In people with HIV who use cannabis compared to those who do not, cannabinoids may help to stabilize the BBB and thereby reduce neuroinflammation.[147, 148] There is a marker to measure this, called neurofilament light, and this marker was reduced in pHIV who used cannabis compared to those who did not.

HIV is not the only virus that has relevance for the BBB-healing properties of cannabinoids. Viruses involved in multiple sclerosis (MS), COVID, mononucleosis (epstein-barr virus: EBV), herpes, and measles can all lead to various degrees of viral encephalitis or brain infection. Cannabinoids and drugs that targeting the CB2R are novel treatments for brain-related impacts of infection. Inflammation in the brain over time will downregulate neurosteroids, leading to depression and anxiety and treating neurological aspects of infection and inflammation is an imperative for health of the body/mind.

Currently the leftover effects (sequelae) of COVID-19 infection have left many of those who were infected with post-acute neurological symptoms of infection, whether or not they had any existing neurologic disease. Fatigue, headaches, memory impairment, and decreased concentration are the most prevalent neurocognitive symptoms. By 6 months post infection, 1/3 of those infected report complete resolution, but about 1/4 of people have worsening of symptoms over time. Addressing the aspects of neuroinflammation and breakdown of the BBB early in infection is important for many viral illnesses.[149]

Case in Point

My patient is a 34-year-old woman who has a primary complaint of chronic joint and myofascial (muscle and deep aching) pain. Her diagnoses include Ehlers-Danlos syndrome (EDS), fibromyalgia, bipolar disorder, history of seizure, and postural orthostatic tachycardic syndrome (POTS). Many of her symptoms started soon after giving birth to her son 2 years earlier. She has a history of mononucleosis in adolescence. She has lingering back, pelvic and shoulder pain prohibiting her from caring for her child and carrying out everyday activities. She scored 8/10 on the Adverse Childhood Experiences (ACEs) scale, having experienced alcoholism and drug abuse by parents, physical harm, emotional abuse, and loss of her mom to cancer. A score on the ACEs questionnaire of 4 or greater is associated with increased risk of many diseases including cancer, addiction, cardiovascular disease, kidney disease and mental health disorders. There is also the potential that there was generational trauma, which means several generations of epigenetic changes due to alterations in the stress response and stress resilience.

She attempted suicide twice. She suffers from complex Post-traumatic stress disorder (cPTSD: a result of incomplete parenting) and reports recurrent nightmares, depression, and panic disorder. Her significant childhood trauma compounds her physical complaints and general health, including overall stress resilience and mental health. By going through the ACEs questionnaire and providing education about the psycho-neurobiological effects of trauma, she is becoming aware of the connection between trauma and health. She is actively engaged in wanting to heal, but has limited financial resources and access to quality healthcare.

She was educated about the role of trauma on systems biology, particularly the role of inflammation on overall health. She was instructed to use vagal toning exercises (abdominal breathing and use of oral mantras) and to discontinue the use of cannabis vape pens, which she says she uses primarily for sleep. The anti-inflammatory effects of cannabis are more likely to occur with low to moderate dosing of cannabis; vape pens exceed this threshold. I prescribed her some plant-based and natural anti-inflammatories: curcumin and palmitoyl-ethanolamine (PEA), high-dose fish oil, N-acetyl cysteine, and vitamin D. I also referred her to an integrative nutritionist for education on anti-inflammatory diet.

Time for a Body Connection Check-in:
First place yourself on the line.

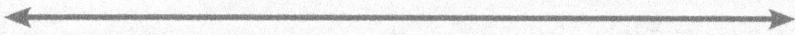

←——————————————————————————————→

++Body Awareness   **Body Detachment++**

For each question below, assess yourself on this scale: not at all, a little bit, sometimes, most of the time, all of the time.

_____ 1. My body feels frozen, as though numb, during uncomfortable situations.

_____ 2. I notice how my body feels when I am angry.

_____ 3. I feel separated from my body.

_____ 4. I listen for information from my body about my emotional state.

_____ 5. It is difficult for me to pay attention to my emotions.

For each time you answered not at all, score a zero; a little bit = 1; some of the time = 2; most of the time = 3; and all of the time = 4. These questions are part of a larger survey on the Scale of Body Connection. How do you score? Statements 1, 3, and 5 assess your body dissociation so a lower score is better. Statements 2 and 4 assess your body attachment, so a higher score is better. Place a mark on the line where you rate yourself and compare this to the first rating that you performed in Chapter 3: Relax. If you are starting to manage stress, and your sleep and digestive function are better, do you think that this has an effect on your body awareness and your self-responsiveness?

She continues to slowly regain her health, with the help of many medical professionals and ongoing trauma therapy. This story highlights the impacts of childhood and/or generational trauma on health. The number and type of ACEs and the timing of the experiences (earlier age) have been shown to be associated with worse health outcomes, including outcomes associated with bipolar disorder.[150] In cases like this, addressing neuroinflammation is imperative for restoring health. Further along in this chapter you will learn more about the postpartum transformation in the immune system that can exacerbate underlying health issues.

Autoimmunity

Auto means self; autoimmunity refers to an attack on the self by the immune system. Autoimmune diseases have increased in recent decades. Rates are the highest where there is increased use of contraception; less incidence of pregnancy is associated with more autoimmune dysfunction. The white blood cells known as T lymphocytes (T-cells) are primarily responsible for ensuring that our immune system does not attack self, or our tissues and proteins. They were named T-cells because they are primarily produced and programmed early in life within a structure called the thymus, a specialized immune organ located in the upper chest behind the breastbone. This mostly happens when we are in the womb and during the early years of life, through adolescence. One of my medical school instructors called it the t cell university, as this is where T-cells are trained in what *is* self and what *is not* self. Simply put, our body can be exposed to an invader (antigen) and the body has something that looks similar to the antigen— a case of molecular mimicry the way autoimmunity is induced.

Once the T-cells are sensitized to the invader and then encounter these self-antigens, antibodies are produced by B-cells (activated by T-cells) that attack our own tissues. There are many types of T-cells, T-cell receptors, and associated cytokines that are known to contribute to the autoimmunity process. THC has been shown to reduce the proliferation of T cells and also to inhibit the synthesis of antibodies by B-cells.[151, 152] The CB2R is thought to be primarily involved in this type of immune cell modulation, as knocking down this receptor in animal studies allows for aggressive T-cell responses, illustrating the homeostatic inhibition of the ECS.[153] However, due to the homeostatic control of the ECS on immunity, while this makes for a nice target for immune-related therapy, the results from animal models of Multiple Sclerosis (MS:using a virus to induce symptoms) show that it is likely not enough to eliminate this disease. Treating animals with cannabinoids has been shown to reduce the severity of disease and also to limit the length of the autoimmune reaction, but not to eliminate it altogether.

This palliation of symptoms, rather than arresting disease, has been highlighted by the drug Sativex (nabiximols), created in Great Britain for use in patients with MS. Use of this oromucosal spray of cannabis extract with THC and CBD in a 1:1 ratio has the potential to help with symptoms of MS (primarily spasticity, pain, bladder control, and sleep), but has not proven to be effective as a disease-modulating drug.[154, 155] While patients with MS may have some short-term benefits on symptoms of the disease, there is little evidence to support that ECS approaches can lead to remyelination of nerves or slow disability in the long term. Using cannabis is not enough to treat or reverse diseases of autoimmunity, as the dose required for immunosuppression can unlikely be achieved. It may, however, be a good immunomodulatory strategy to use in combination with other disease-modifying therapies and integrative health-building approaches.

Hypersensitivity Reactions

This type of immune reaction is due to the combination of genetics that predispose some people to react to environmental conditions. It is a reaction of being hypersensitive to external stimuli such as fragrances, bee stings, chemicals, or foods. A hypersensitivity reaction can result in either a mild or deadly reaction. An acute hypersensitivity reaction requires the use of injected epinephrine to stop the process. Mild hypersensitivity reactions of the skin may respond to use of topical cannabis. It is possible to have sensitivities to foods or substances that do not involve a full-blown hypersensitivity reaction. Elimination diets and cleaning up the environment you live in, including cleaning and body care products, may be in order. Calming mast cells activity is also needed. In this situation, mast cell activation syndrome may be diagnosed and treated.

Cannabis Use and the Immune Response

Since the early 1970s, soon after THC was isolated, there has been investigation into the immune effects of cannabis. THC was shown to affect immune modulators in animals and in blood cells from humans who smoked cannabis. These effects were not confirmed by other investigators, however, and until the cannabinoid receptors were discovered and found to be expressed on immune cells in 1995, research into these effects slowed.[156] Studies of immune cells from the lungs of cannabis smokers demonstrated an altered production of cytokines and lack of production of nitric oxide, consistent with what would be considered immunosuppression. The ECS has a large role in lung function, including making sure we have enough oxygen to survive, breathing rate and modulating the immune system in the lungs.[157]

In mouse models of pneumonia, mice treated with THC (100 mcg, given intravenously) died due to lack of T-cell proliferation when rechallenged with the bacteria. This suggested negative effects of THC on adaptive immunity (the defensive team) in humans, but this has not yet been substantiated. There have been concerns around cannabis use in cancer about inhibiting the immune function, response to viral infection (such as HIV), but these have yet to be substantiated in large groups of people. The suppression of normal immune responses has not been clearly demonstrated to increase susceptibility to or promote infections, diseases, or lead to the progression of cancers in humans.

For potential immunomodulation, similar to other scenarios, there could be a biphasic effect of THC on the immune response, but the doses shown to clearly inhibit immune responses in animals (30–150 mg/kg) is unlikely to be achieved in humans. If immunosuppression was a reality in humans using cannabis, then these immune-modulatory effects of cannabinoids on inflammatory and autoimmune disorders would be more apparent. The most relevant exception is smoking (burning) of cannabis, which clearly has effects on lung health and the immune component of the respiratory system. To avoid this scenario, a harm-reduction approach is to use a plant vaporizer (not a vape pen) as the harsh concentration of chemicals in vape pens has similar damaging effects as smoking.

Therapeutic dosing of oral ingestion of cannabis products is also unlikely to induce immune suppression, although there can be individual variations that can impact the effects. Interestingly, although cannabinoids appear to exert a small degree of immune suppression when innate immune cells are activated, this does not seem to be the case when immune cells are resting or not reacting to an invader.

Body/Mind Interface 4

Therapies such as mindfulness-based meditation, yoga, tai chi, and qigong have been shown to have profound beneficial effects on the immune system. These therapies are considered to be multidimensional in that they bring together physical activity and behavioral activity to promote stress reduction and relaxation. By regulating our emotional responses to stress, we can influence our immune systems! We have a lot of power using our body/mind. Inflammatory markers such as C-reactive protein (a non-specific marker of inflammation) and pro-inflammatory cytokines (IL-6, TNF-alpha, IFN-gamma), and also improve function of lymphocytes and responses to vaccines. For these effects, practicing one of these techniques at least once per week, 60–180 minutes per week; engaging in consistent practice of these activities—would be ideal! Body-mind therapies can reduce markers of inflammation.[158] You can use the Scale of Body Connection to measure changes in your own sensitivity to your internal state, and you can also employ body work, such as massage and other somatic therapies, to enhance your interoception (use the Scale of Body Connection to monitor yourself). A happy mood builds a flourishing immune system.

Women's Health

Fertility

Women face many unique challenges. Regarding fertility, the challenge is how to grow a genetically distinct human in their bodies without their immune systems rejecting the fetus as a foreign object. This is a complicated strategy that enables the body to fight off pathogens without endangering the fetus; here again there is a role for the ECS. We established that the ECS is present in all reproductive tissues. During ovulation, the presence of progesterone inhibits the production of AEA in the lining of the uterus (one of the places where AEA is the highest in all of the reproductive tissues) by upregulating the enzyme FAAH, which breaks down AEA. Uterine levels apparently need to be *low* in order for a fertilized egg to be able to implant in the uterus (a process called decidualization that changes a layer of mucous membrane). Low levels of FAAH and associated high levels of AEA are associated with both infertility and less chance of success at in vitro fertilization (IVF). At the beginning of pregnancy, the immune system ramps up in a response similar to that of reacting to a wound, necessary for the fertilized egg to, in effect, damage the uterine lining and establish a blood supply.

Pregnancy is an immune privileged situation where immune responses tend to be slowed in some respects, as there is less histamine release due to mast cell inactivation. There are increases in the monocyte population of cells, but they may be the anti-inflammatory, repair-type of monocytes (macrophages), and this profile shifts over the course of a pregnancy. A specialized type of natural killer (NK) cells are found in the placental decidua, and are important for helping establish the blood supply to the placenta. The killer cells are not on a search-and-destroy mission as they usually are. The decidua is helping to protect the embryo, as a barrier, from being attacked by maternal immune cells. The immune system is in a new adapted state for pregnancy. It returns to homeostasis when pregnancy ends.

Postpartum Immune Changes and Depression

T-cell numbers don't change in pregnancy, but the shifting of ratios of cell types results in improvement in symptoms of some autoimmune disorders, such as rheumatoid arthritis and MS.[159] This shift occurring, called a TH1 to TH2 shift, is typically a rapidly resolving situation, by 4 weeks postpartum. This rapid shift back to homeostatic immunity is a major player in PPD, a situation where brain inflammation may need to be treated.

PPD is a normal, not uncommon experience also known as the 'baby blues'. This experience can be different for everyone who experiences it due to many factors. When you think you should be feeling happy about your new little one, instead there may be tears and depressed mood starting anywhere from 3 to 10 days after birth. It's a result of shifting hormones, sleep deprivation, and the emergence of a new you that includes a body that may seem unfamiliar to you and a new role. PPD is 100% treatable, so know that with the appropriate care and support, you can recover without feeling alone or sad or maybe even hopeless. You are not an unfit mother for having this experience!

Symptoms of PPD can include feeling detached from your baby, inability to function, feeling irritable or sad, depression, and even thoughts of harming oneself or the baby. Functionally, these symptoms can occur anytime during your baby's first year of life, but are sometimes more prolonged. There is no shame in seeking help if you feel this way because, left untreated, this syndrome is scary for some women and at the very least steals the joy around the arrival of a new being.

Here is a deeper dive into the neurochemical underpinnings of PPD. The placenta is steroidogenic and so all steroid hormones plummet initially after birth as the ovaries and other steroid machinery regroup and stabilize. Pregnenolone is called the mother hormone. It is the compound made when cholesterol is taken through its first chemical transformation at the mitochondrial level. Pregnenolone then is stored as a sulfated form or can be converted to DHEA-sulfate (DHEA-s).*

Both of these chemicals are reservoirs (easier to transport in the blood) for making other steroid hormones such as estradiol, testosterone, and cortisol

---

* DHEA is a steroid hormone called dehydroepiandrosterone, a precursor molecule for androgens and estrogens and DHEAs is a storage form, ready to be called to action.

(estrone and cholesterol are also found in sulfated forms). Mutations in the steroid sulfatase (STS) enzyme can reduce the activity of converting these compounds back to the free or available form. These mutations can predispose people to having more depression and more PPD.

Even outside of pregnancy, people with these genetics may live with elevated levels irritability, low energy, psychological distress, and manic symptoms as well as differences with respect to sleeping patterns. This information highlights the importance of the neurosteroid allopregnanolone, made from pregnenolone. Our mother hormone is therefore effective at helping the GABA receptor to be more receptive to GABA, a neuroinhibitory neurotransmitter. This leads to less anxiety and depression.[160]

BOX 4.2   ENDOCRINE DISRUPTORS: High toxic doses of chemicals are not necessarily required to disrupt our biochemistry. Low doses of chemicals over time (chronic low dose) are just as dangerous. Our endogenous hormones are at low dose and have strong effects even at low concentration. The same is true for synthetic compounds that can interfere with making steroids and with the protein receptors activated by them: bisphenol A (found in plastics); phthalates—used in softer plastics (children's toys, cosmetics, and personal care products); insecticides inhibit conversion of testosterone to estrogen (non-organic foods); parabens are pro-estrogenic (a preservative found in cosmetics and sunscreen); phenols—weakly estrogenic (detergents). *You can search for endocrine disruptors in your body care and cleaning products at EWR.org.*

As mentioned in Chapter Relax, the chemical analog to the neuro-steroid allopregnanolone (brexanolone or Zulresso, currently given as an IV infusion), was approved by the FDA in 2019 to treat PPD. This medication will soon be available as an oral tablet approved for PPD. There are supplement forms of bioidentical pregnenolone and DHEA, but the problem is that due to enzyme regulation, there is no assurance that either of these will be directed to the pathway where they are most needed.

Other means of addressing the neuroinflammation that can occur postpartum, due to the rapid switching of the immune function, include supporting the immune system before and pregnancy. Supplementation with vitamin

D is in order as it is difficult to raise blood levels through diet alone.[161] Low vitamin D levels have been associated with higher PPD symptoms. Vitamin A is another important nutrient for immune health. Other sources for fighting neuroinflammation include eating an anti-inflammatory diet, using natural and botanical anti-inflammatories, optimizing sleep, nutrition, and mental health before conceiving, and seeking out and eliminating endocrine disruptors (see Box 4.2). Unfortunately, we can't change our genetics. But we *can* work to optimize the genetics, epigenetically, that we were born with.

There are certainly many variables that can contribute to both the inability to get pregnant and the inflammatory postpartum picture. Notably, women without social support, in abusive relationships, or financially stressed will have higher activation of the HPA axis and more inflammation than without these scenarios. As preventives for those who may have fertility issues, not using THC or CBD when trying to get pregnant may give your immune system the best chance of doing its implantation job well. CBD has been reported to inhibit the FAAH enzyme and thereby theoretically raise AEA levels, so using CBD (hemp) could impair the critical processes occurring immunologically at the site of implantation.[162] The CBD dose at which this could occur is unknown, but 400 mg/day for 28 days was not shown to increase AEA when given to people who had cannabis use disorder.[163] It is unlikely that the low doses of CBD available in most products would interfere with reproductive function.

Autoimmune Diseases in Women

Women are 3 time as likely as men to develop an autoimmune disease such as MS, rheumatoid arthritis (RA), systemic lupus, and Hashimoto thyroiditis. This is thought to be due to the expression of 2 X chromosomes and the genes linked to these chromosomes, HLA receptor variability in the immune system, and the contribution of steroid hormones.* This is

---

* HLA is human leukocyte antigen receptors and is controlled by genetics. This gene encodes for cells to present antigen on their surface to present them to T-cells. There are some known HLA mutations that are related to specific inflammatory diseases such as multiple sclerosis, psoriasis, rheumatoid arthritis, and type 1 diabetes.

evidenced partially by the onset of autoimmune diseases in women shortly after puberty and the remission of symptoms during pregnancy or after menopause (highest incidence between ages of 10–40). For instance, in MS there is demyelination of nerves due to loss of self-tolerance to myelin, the insulator of nerves that allows for neurotransmission. Immune alterations taking place during pregnancy induce a protective immune shift in cases of a cell-mediated disease (the TH1 to TH2 shift mentioned earlier) with a 70% reduction in the MS relapse rate. This may be due to estrogenic effects on T-regulatory cells or immune-protective effects of high levels of progesterone in pregnancy.

There is a sex bias for autoimmunity, perhaps because women have stronger immune responses in general than men, giving us a survival advantage— but at a cost. During embryogenesis, receiving two X chromosomes or being female, can lead to overexpression of some immune-related genes and micro RNAs. (mRNAs are genetic material, but they do not code for protein expression like genes do.)

This highlights the role of a well-functioning and toned endocannabinoid system to help with over-proliferation of T-cells, appropriate activation of cannabinoid receptors, and not downregulating the system by overuse of THC (high-potency products and high frequency of use). Both the endogenous system and phytocannabinoids such as THC and CBD, and maybe other understudied minor cannabinoids, may eventually be exploited to help treat autoimmunity.

Endometriosis is a condition that is inflammatory, not yet classified as an autoimmune disease, and affects up to 20% of cycling women. Endometrial cells are the lining of the uterus which thickens after ovulation in mammals, forming an epithelial, mucus layer for implanting a fertilized egg. When progesterone rises after ovulation, this normally triggers cell death for this layer, which is released during menstruation and then starts rebuilding (with some birth control methods, this lining becomes dormant). Estrogen stimulates the proliferation of this lining. When these epithelial cells migrate out of the uterine environment, it causes a chronic inflammatory disease associated with pain during menstruation and chronic pelvic pain during the rest of the cycle. Infertility is often associated with endometriosis.

Why do these cells not stay put and wreak havoc? One theory is thought to be due to retrograde menstruation, where the cells migrate through the fallopian tubes adhering to the wall of the lining of the abdomen (peritoneum) and there they proliferate. Another theory is that a sex-hormone-dependent mechanism transforms peritoneal cells into an epithelial type. It has also been considered to be an autoimmune disease because of association with presence of autoantibodies.

Normally, NK cells would scavenge these out-of-context cells and a decrease of NK cell function may also be involved. Endometriosis has other features of autoimmunity including tissue damage, immune-related spontaneous abortion, abnormal T-cell activation and other immune cell dysfunction. Left untreated, this disease can be associated with the development of reproductive cancers, such as uterine cancer. Balancing estrogen and progesterone is an important part of helping to treat endometriosis. Pain benefit may be found with ibuprofen (reducing prostaglandin production). Cannabis can be a helpful tool for chronic pelvic pain and add a layer of anti-inflammatory protection. There is some evidence, not yet strong in humans, that cannabinoids may contribute to the taming of B-cells, to slow antibody production, or switch their phenotypes in a beneficial manner. PEA is also anti-inflammatory and has been used to calm mast cells, which are inflammatory and pain mediators in endometriosis tissue.[164] Boosting the ECS function in general and specifically targeting CB2 can reduce proliferation of cells and promote anti-inflammatory pathways (suggestions following at the end of the chapter).

Fibromyalgia is a chronic condition associated with tenderness and pain across the body. There used to be no diagnosis for this, and women, twice as likely as men to suffer from this condition, were often told it was a somatic disorder. A somatic disorder is one that is mental but manifests in the body when there is no other organic cause to explain it. There are diagnostic criteria for fibromyalgia and evidence emerging that it may be another autoimmune condition. This would make sense as it tends to run in families. Cannabis can help to ease the pain and also help to address the associated sleep disturbance that many people with this diagnosis have. There is also likely immune modulating benefit for this patient population.

With estrogen loss associated with menopause (more in Forget), a bothersome or sometimes debilitating side effect is arthralgia or joint pain—arthritis. I bought some wild-caught herring, because it contains more omega-3 fatty acids (FA) than either salmon or mackerel (but not as much as sardines) and I like to use food as preventive medicine. Arthragia-associated stiffness, joint swelling, pain, and fatigue are symptoms that Omega-3s can help! Sometimes it can be better or worse after movement. More severe forms of joint pain are osteoarthritis (degeneration) and RA (inflammatory and autoimmune). Specifically, RA symptoms can flare with triggers such as stress, too much activity, environmental factors, or sometimes with no clear cause. The goal is to control joint pain and try to keep it in remission. Severe pain may need to be treated with joint injections.

Why omega-3 supplementation? Our body does not make FAs with the first double bond at the number 3 position (why they are called omega-3s) so they are essential nutrients we have to get from diet. These omega-3 compounds are immunomodulatory, as they can limit or modulate inflammatory responses, and have been shown to do so in arthritis. The 2 major omega-3s are docosahexaenoic acid (DHA: a 22-carbon chain FA) and eicosapentaenoic acid (EPA:a 20-carbon chain FA). Endocannabinoids also have 20 carbons; this class is known as eicosanoids. Arachidonic acid also has 20 carbons, but is an omega-6 FA, the starting compound for endocannabinoids. Dietarily, it is healthful to have at least 1 gram of omega-3s for every 4 grams of omega-6; we need about 2 grams of omega 3 daily.

Will eating more omega-3s (or taking a supplement of fish oil) deplete our ECBs? The simple answer is no, because there is a class of omega-3 endocannabinoids called DHA-EA and DHG (the 22-carbon form) and EPA-EA and EPG (the 20-carbon form that is not omega-6). DHA-EA does not act at the cannabinoid receptors with high potency (10-20x less potent) but EPA-EA is still potent at CB1R and CB2R. Therefore, the amount of omega-3 FA being stored in the cell membrane can shift our endocannabinoids. The cyclooxygenase enzymes (COX1/COX2) come into play as does another enzyme called lipoxygenase (LOX). When the omega-6 endocannabinoids (AEA and 2AG) are broken down by COX and LOX, the result can be pro-inflammatory molecules, because arachidonic acid (AA) is generally associated with these bad lipid signalers. This is how ibuprofen works, by blocking COX-2 and therefore inhibiting the compounds made.

By supplementing dietary DHA and EPA there is a decrease in arachidonic acid (AA) so less fuel for COX and LOX to make pro-inflammatory compounds. When these enzymes are used to break down DHA-EA and EPA-EA or DHG or EPG, the compounds made are called resolvins, protectins, and maresin, which help to quench inflammation![165] These have been shown to reduce pain in postmenopausal women who were supplemented with omega-3 FAs.[166,167] This approach can also be helpful not only in arthritis but also in the autoimmune disease lupus, improving bone mineral density, anxiety, and depression, and for brain health, as we will see in Chapter 5: Forget.[ ]

Vaginal tone, the Bladder and Infections

Like the gut, our urinary tract and vagina have a microbiome that is distinct from the one in the gut. These areas are not sterile as once thought, and the bug community living there is involved in the health of our bladder, ureters, and vagina. Anywhere the inside world meets the outside world, there is a coexisting community of microbes. As a result of monthly fluctuations in hormones, this community can shift and change over time. Imbalances in this collection of critters is associated with bacterial vaginosis, yeast infections, interstitial cystitis, overactive bladder, and urinary incontinence. Plant cannabinoids are anti-microbial as are the terpenes, so the essential oil of cannabis is a potential means for helping with bacterial balance in the genito-urinary tract.[168] For mild infections, a suppository made with the cannabis essential oil (this could be from a CO_2 extraction where the terpenoids are retained) can be inserted vaginally at bedtime. You will want to lie down so the oil does not leak out. The cannabinoids don't tend to get into circulation or make you high when used in a suppository form. (results may vary!) Underlying chronic genitourinary infections are typically hormone imbalances, so working with a qualified provider to balance hormones is the means to treat the cause. Use of probiotics for the genitourinary tract can also be helpful.

Naturopathic/Integrative/Functional Approaches

You can tone your endocannabinoid system on a daily basis by using compounds that are known to be activators of the CB2 receptor. Here are some dietary CB2 agonists:

- PEA is a relative of AEA, in the endocannabinoid family of compounds, and is also made in our body. It inhibits a receptor called PPAR-alpha, where it acts as an anti-inflammatory compound. It is found in our diet in egg yolks, peanuts, organ meats, olive oil, soy lecithin, and edamame. It can also be taken as a supplement, but may not be stable in stomach acid, so needs a special preparation to make it past the stomach acid. This may be helpful for inflammation in endometriosis.[ ]

- ß-caryophyllene is an aromatic compound found in cannabis that is a CB2R full agonist with quite high affinity for the receptor. It is also found in clove, oregano, cinnamon, and black pepper, so spice up your food![169]

- The Cruciferae family of vegetables contains indole-3 carbinol (I3C), which our body converts to 3,3 diindolylmethane (DIM). In addition to modulating enzymes that help us to detox DIM is also a CB2 partial agonist This includes broccoli, brussels sprouts, collard greens, cabbages, mustard, kales, bok choy, cauliflower, and others.[170, 171] Eat these every day!

- Cannabichromene (CBC) is an intermediate cannabinoid found in the cannabis plant but not usually in high concentration. It has been found to act as an agonist at CB2R, but what human dose might be therapeutic is unknown.

- Cannabigerol (CBG) is the mother cannabinoid that the cannabis plant uses to make other cannabinoid compounds first identified in 1964. There is typically little of this natural product at the harvest time of the plant, but breeders are knocking down the genes for making CBD and THC so as to leave CBG in the plant in a higher amount. This cannabinoid does not have psychoactive effects like THC, and may be a weak partial agonist at CB2R and antagonist at CB1R. It is not yet known what dose in humans could be beneficial as an anti-inflammatory or other purposes.[172]

Sleep

The importance of regularly timed sleep on a circadian schedule, with good sleep architecture and adequate amount of sleep, cannot be understated! If you have not yet made any sleep adjustments, I hope that this section on inflammation and immunity might give you more ambition to adjust your habits, or get the help you need in order to have healthy sleep.

Terpene

Limonene has been shown to have potential anticancer activity preclinically. It has been shown to inhibit cell proliferation and is safe and tolerable for humans for ingestion.[173] It is highly bioavailable via dry vaping in chemotypes that contain amounts of this compound. Sour Diesel, Gelato, and Tahoe OG Kush are some chemotypes that may have significant amounts of limonene.[174] However, plant names are not a great indicator of the chemical composition. Ask to see the laboratory analysis and breakdown of the terpene profile.

Allostatic Load

Triglycerides, blood pressure, heart rate variability, calprotectin, C-reactive protein, erythrocyte sedimentation rate, cytokines, and procalcitonin are measures of AL. Serial hormone testing across a monthly cycle can help point to specifics of your hormonal cycle, how you metabolize hormones and targeting the means to balance them.

Herbal Allies

All medicinal mushrooms are shown to have immunomodulatory effects. Rotating these mushrooms or taking a combination of them during times of stress, when immunity is impacted, or when sick or fighting cancer is a food-as-medicine approach. Many of these can be used in your diet:

shiitake, maitake, and oyster mushrooms can be found in grocery stores, along with the common agaricus (black button).

Ganoderma lucidum, or Reishi mushroom, is a highly respected botanical from Chinese medicine. It has been hailed as the mushroom of the immortals for its use to preserve health, support mental calmness, and promote longevity for thousands of years in China. Reishi is considered to be a broad-acting immune modulating mushroom, which has a wider spectrum of action compared to some other botanicals researched. Its potential benefits include decreasing cell proliferation, anti-allergenic, antiviral, antitumor, anti-inflammatory, antioxidant, and hepato-protective effects.[175]

Anti-inflammatories

Zingiber officinale: Ginger has been shown to inhibit activation and migration of immune cells, decrease pro-inflammatory cytokines, inhibit COX enzymes (what ibuprofen does), and provide antioxidant activity. Fresh-juiced ginger (added to pineapple tastes great!) added to soups, kombucha, soup, and teas, whether sweet or savory.[176]

Echinacea angustifolia: This herb is native to North America and was widely used by Native American populations. Extracts have been described as being immunostimulatory, and anti-inflammatory but investigations into the use of echinacea to treat viral infections have been inconclusive. Native Americans were said to have used it for snake bites. Echinacea contains alkylamide compounds[177, 178] found in number of botanical medicines, considered to be CB_2 partial agonists. These compounds have been shown to inhibit TNFα and to inhibit AEA reuptake. Alkylamides are considered to be cannabimimetic, and modulate TNFa (pro-inflammatory cytokine) expression for immunomodulatory effects.[179] Specifically, this class of compounds has been described to act through the CB2R, primarily expressed on immune cells, but also in the dorsal root ganglia and involved in pain signaling.[180] Alkylamides may also play a role in relief of anxiety through the anti-inflammatory action at CB2 receptor.[181] Compounds from the echinacea root were also reported to inhibit FAAH, thereby increasing AEA levels.[182] It does not taste particularly great, and alcohol is needed to extract the lipophilic alkylamides, so you might want to use this plant in a capsule or a glycerine preparation. These compounds are also in *achillea millefolium* (yarrow), *spilanthes acmella, zanthoxylum piperitum* (Japanese prickly ash), and *capsicum* fruits (peppers).

Tripterygium wilfordii: Thundergod vine is traditional to Chinese medicine and contains celastrol, reported to be a CB2R agonist. This plant has been used for arthritis and autoimmune disease, but there are some safety concerns about toxicity to the liver from the presence of pyridine alkaloids (also found in *kava methysticum*).

Piper methysticum: Kava kava contains yangonin, a kavalactone compound has pharmacological activity at the CB1R, with moderate affinity, which can explain some of the effects of kava.[183] *P. longum* (a related species) has been used as an analgesic, immune-modulator, aphrodisiac, or emmenagogue to treat respiratory or gastrointestinal disorders, post-partum hemorrhage, epilepsy, diabetes, and RA.[184] Among the bioactive molecules are piperamides, shown to have analgesic, antidepressant, anti-inflammatory, and hepatoprotective effects.

Piper sp. (black and long pepper): Specifically, guineesine, a piperamide, inhibits the reuptake of the endocannabinoid AEA with nanomolar affinity, and also shown to have cannabimimetic effects.[ ] Additionally, *Piper sp.* fruits also contain significant amounts of the sesquiterpene beta-caryophyllene, which is a CB2R agonist.[ ]

Curcuma longa: Curcumin is the active ingredient in the spice turmeric (common in yellow curry mixes) and is reported to act as an anti-inflammatory by inhibiting cyclooxygenase 2 (COX-2) and lipoxygenase (LOX) enzymes, which mostly produce pro-inflammatory compounds and inducible nitric oxide synthase (a ROS).

Camelia sinensis: Phenylpropanoids such as epigallocatechin-3-gallate (EGCG) is found in both green and black tea as well as other foods and is a low-potency binder of the CB1R.[185]

Eugenia caryophyllata, or clove, contains a high content of beta-caryophyllene (BCP), a sesquiterpene alkene and CB2 receptor full agonist (K_i 155 nM) dietary cannabinoid considered to have a wide safety margin and to be nontoxic.[,186] Cannabimimetic foods, or compounds that are secondary metabolites in plants, and play unrecognized roles in human physiology and biochemistry. Specific to the CB2 receptor is the homeostatic role of the ECS in limiting inflammation.[,187] BCP is also found in *Cannabis spp.* essential oil, shown to be effective at reducing neuropathic pain, and is approved as a food additive by the FDA.[188] BCP is available from vegetables and spices, typically in doses of around 10 mg, but will vary with diet.

Food/Diet/Nutrition

A simple, 2–3 times per day hack for addressing inflammation is to eat an anti-inflammatory diet. The Dietary Inflammatory Index is one way to assess how you are eating, and accessing a nutritionist can guide you in evaluating your score. The Mediterranean diet or the Whole30 plan are two great ways to get started on improving your food choices. It can take a lot of willpower to change habits. Don't underestimate the power of food as medicine. Until relatively recently, plants were all we had to keep us alive! Getting back to nature is the most sustainable way for us to live.

Time-restricted eating and/or intermittent fasting and caloric restriction are all means of reducing inflammation, such as for cardiovascular risk. Just giving the body a break from digesting and taking in fewer calories can help reduce oxidative stress and inflammatory markers in the blood. Fasting releases some anti-inflammatory and repair macrophages into the blood circulation, and these types of macrophages help to repair tissues, resulting in less joint pain. It is suggested that these practices occur in the long term (1 year) for optimal results.

Flavonoids: These compounds are found in all fresh fruits and vegetables, and cover a wide range of compounds. Many of these are simple to remember because they are the colors of our food. Eating a rainbow daily is the task! Here is a breakdown on some of the colors, antioxidant compounds, and foods containing them.

- Carotenoids: Deep red, yellow, and orange color—butternut/acorn squash, eggs, butter, sweet potato, pumpkin, cantaloupe, mango, greens

- Lycopene: Red—tomato, strawberry, papaya, guava, watermelon
- Anthocyanins: Deep purple and blue-red cabbage, cranberry, blackberry
- Ellagitannins: Berries of all kinds and pomegranate
- Catechins: Dark chocolate
- Resveratrol: Found in red grapes (particularly the skins)
- Astaxanthin: Found in salmon, trout, krill, shrimp, and crayfish

Yoga/Chakra

The first chakra, muladhara, is known as the root chakra, located in the base of the spine. It is associated with the color red and our connection to the earth and governs security, stability, and sensuality. It is related to our physical survival. A yoga practice in general will boost immune health, due to the stress-resolving, circulatory, and breathwork components.

The legs up the wall or viparita karani pose is simple, relaxing, and rejuvenating. Any seated yoga posture is associated with this chakra. The mula bandha is the root lock in which the muscles at the center of the perineum (midway between the anus and genitals) are tightly contracted. To engage with this, start with slow gentle contraction, pulling the perineum up to a maximum point, hold briefly, and then lower back down. You can increase the strength of the contraction to your tolerance. This bandha is done with breathwork (I suggest an instructor skilled in yoga) and is thought to have many benefits including stabilizing and calming, calming sympathetic arousal, urogenital function harmony, and benefit for self-awareness.

CHAPTER 5:

Forget

When I am an old woman I shall wear purple
With a red hat which doesn't go, and doesn't suit me.
And I shall spend my pension on brandy and summer gloves
And satin sandals, and say we've no money for butter.
I shall sit down on the pavement when I'm tired
And gobble up samples in shops and press alarm bells
And run my stick along the public railings
And make up for the sobriety of my youth.
I shall go out in my slippers in the rain
And pick flowers in other people's gardens
And learn to spit.

—Jenny Joseph, English poet

Overview of Memory

My local surf spot is a beach break which means that the breaking wave is due to the underwater part of the wave dragging on the shallow sandy beach bottom, often causing the wave to break all at once or close out. When a wave closes out it doesn't offer a non-vertical wall where surfers ride so they not great from the surfing perspective. This situation is however a highly fluctuating situation that depends on the wave size, tide, swell direction (a swell is a wind-generated series of waves), and time of year.

I'm told that in the 1950s the area was all rock and reef, no sandy beach. The real estate and tourist industries partnered with the city to build the beaches by dredging sand from the bay and hauling it out to the beachfront areas. This process entirely changed the surf. Instead of waves dragging on the corner of a rock pile and gently peeling away (a reef break), they are more likely to close out. The wave architecture changes according to the season. In 2023, a series of atmospheric rivers brought the biggest swell California has seen in 10 years. In addition to king tides (exceptionally high and low tides due to gravitational pull of the moon), much of the beach is eroded and rock-covered, as it likely was 70 years ago.

Big waves/tide suck the sand out in the winter, leaving their seasonal mark. Then, amazingly, in the summer, the sand gets washed back in by swells coming from the south. How a beach will settle changes year-to-year, tide-to-tide, swell-to-swell, and based on the direction from which the swell and winds come. This malleability of the coast and surf conditions are comparable to the process of plasticity in the brain.

Our brains are plastic, meaning that neuronal wiring is flexible and able to be reshaped or reprogrammed. Our brain comes with a built-in ability to reorganize itself—structure, function, and neuronal connections—changing its activity based on external and internal signals. Plasticity is a hallmark of the human brain, allowing us to develop highly complex cognitive skills. We experience plasticity with learning and memory when we are in rapidly changing environments (surfing!), in conversation, and if we have brain disease (such as TBI or PD). Plasticity is a physiologic change that can last for short or long periods of time. Interestingly, humans may have an evolutionary advantage by having both neuronal and immune systems that are highly plastic, allowing for a super intelligent sensing of, and ability to adapt to, our internal and external environments—known as neuroimmune symbiosis.

Endocannabinoids regulate synaptic plasticity, very generally, by inhibiting neurotransmitter release. This was first discovered in the hippocampus, the brain's memory pantry, a structure deep in the temporal lobe of the brain. It is an area richly supplied with the ECS, highly innervated by acetylcholine (ACh) receptors, a neurotransmitter system that is associated with disorders such as AD and epilepsy.[189]

A pioneer of modern neuroscience from Spain, Santiago Ramón y Cajál studied neurons and in 1892 was the first to suggest that we could augment our brain capacity by increasing the connections between neurons. By 1900, the links between nerves and chemicals as signaling agents were being made. The space between nerve endings, where nerves communicate, is the synapse, the prime real estate where short-term plasticity occurs. Short-term plasticity is rapid, bidirectional, and reversible—modulating the strength of connections caused by the release of neurotransmitters: occurring in tens-to-hundreds of milliseconds. For comparison, the blink of your eye takes about three one hundredths of a second. Sodium fuels all of this!

The ECS Role in Neurotransmission

Soon after THC was first isolated, a classic assay was designed for testing the effects of cannabinoids in animals. A tetrad of THC effects[190] was first described in the lab of researcher Billy Martin, who studied addiction and how drugs affect the brain; the tetrad measures:

1. Body temperature: a drop in body temperature
2. Catalepsy: immobility when hung from a bar
3. Hypomobility: decreased movement around the animal enclosure
4. Analgesia: increased threshold to pain (could tolerate a higher heat applied to the paw)

These effects were first thought to be occurring through binding the opioid receptor, but as research on the ECS grew, enabled by the isolation of THC, early researchers such as Dr. Martin discovered that the ECS was the target. Eventually it was learned that the ECS was intimately involved in brain plasticity.

As previously mentioned, there are 2 types of plasticity: both short term and long term. Short-term plasticity modulates the probability for neurotransmitter release from vesicles at the synapse, a process dependent upon calcium flowing in at the presynaptic neuron after sodium has flowed in. (There may be as many as 1,000 contacts being made at the postsynaptic neuron—at least tens to hundreds).[191] This calcium influx is under the control of the ECS through CB1R signaling. THC, similarly to endocannabinoids, activates CB1R, thereby closing calcium channels and concluding the neurotransmitter release (GABA, glutamate, acetylcholine, dopamine). In addition, there are other mediators of plasticity such as the NMDA receptor, brain-derived neurotropic factor (BDNF), nerve growth factor (NGF), hormones, nutrition, and changes in gene expression that have roles in mediating plasticity. One takeaway message is that what we do and what we are exposed to influences our brain on a daily basis. This may be beneficial or harmful.

Long-term plasticity is considered to be a primary mechanism for learning and memory and can be modulated by increasing or decreasing protein receptors at the synapse and by regulating release of neurotransmitters. Strengthening (potentiation) or weakening (depression) of the synaptic activity are hallmarks of long-term plasticity. The process whereby synapses are weakened (long-term depression) is considered to be a fundamental mechanism by which we change behaviors, by way of neural circuitry. Endocannabinoids are required as a part of this process occurring in neurons whether they are excitatory (glutamate) or inhibitory (GABA), but the regulatory effects of the ECS are not exclusive to signaling through these two transmitters. It is through ECS. machinery that THC alters learning and memory, executive function and perception. Generally, binding of CB1R is considered to have inhibitory effects on neuronal excitability, which is important for fine-tuning plasticity. Due to biphasic effects, the opposite can occur with high dose of THC. This is due to the affinity of the CB1R at different types of neurotransmitter receptors with glutamate having the highest affinity and GABA having a much lower affinity for THC. This way as the THC dose increases, by binding at GABA terminals at high dose, there is an inhibition of inhibition: excitation.

G-protein coupled receptor (GPCR) is the class of protein receptors that CBRs belong to. They perform their actions by use of what are known as second messengers. This is different from ion channels, which open in response to stimuli allowing ions (charged atoms) either into or out of the cell. Ions typically induce a rapid response (milliseconds), while GPCRs are involved in slower (seconds to minutes time frame). More lasting changes occur by inducing genes at the nucleus. Both of these types of receptors (metabotropic or ionotropic) interact with neurotransmitters and while CBR are GPCRs, they also regulate ion flow (notably calcium and potassium).

The TRPV1 receptor is a calcium channel and considered to be in the ECS family. Serotonin and dopamine receptors are other types of GPCRs. To further complicate matters, these GPCRs can join (in a form called a heterodimer) to induce signaling that neither receptor can accomplish alone.[192] This is the beauty of conservation in the human body. In fact, CBR1 agonists alone do not participate in long-term plasticity without other players. One of them is NMDA (discussed later with relationship to ketamine). The cannabinoid receptors are notable for heterodimerizing, not surprising given the promiscuity of the ECS across tissues and functions in homeostasis.

The ECS Provides That We Forget

"It's a poor sort of memory that only works backwards."
–The White Queen in Lewis Carroll's *Alice in Wonderland*)

Fine-tuning of the ECS, with a special emphasis on CB1R, underlies the important functions of learning and memory (forgetting or not forgetting). This ECS-regulated process is one that allows us to take in (learn), store (consolidation), recall (retrieval), and modify (reconsolidate) our experiences or forget them. How we perceive our environment, as well as how it changes, is basic to survival. And you already have learned about how our ECS outside of the brain is geared for this survival from other aspects (metabolism, sleeping, relaxing, and protecting).

An interesting thing to note is that the action of ECBs at the CBRs varies, due to different chemical structures. This means that various cannabinoid compounds (agonists) may not always affect these ECS processes exactly the same way as the ECBs. For instance, THC is considered to be a partial agonist at CB1R while AEA and 2AG are full agonists—the structure of the chemical and how/where it binds to the protein receptor dictates the function of the protein. THC elicits distinct effects on working memory, what most people refer to as being stoned. We don't feel stoned all of the time, despite the fact that we have ECBs in our system and binding the CB1R.

Memory

Effects on learning, retaining what is learned into memory, and being able to recall what we learned can be affected for periods of time longer than just the time a person feels high (known as the acute effects: all effects are dose-related and results may vary). One form of memory is called working memory—the type limited to a short period of time, such as remembering ingredients in a recipe as you are assembling it. Working memory can be impaired by THC use but not by the action of ECBs at their normal levels in blood or tissue. By inhibiting FAAH, the level of AEA can be raised in the brain. This has not been shown to be detrimental to working memory, at least in mice it was not.[193] The THC-associated impairment is a form of mind wandering or zoning out (my old friend calls this a whiteout). Meta-cognition—thinking about what one is thinking, or planning and monitoring of oneself and our performance—can be like reflecting on or evaluating our level of confidence in our actions (Did I add the right amount of salt?).[194]

When learning something new there are changes in neuronal connections: 1) growth and pruning of dendrites and 2) growth of axons. Important in the growth of the dendritic spiny projections is a factor called BDNF, a neurotropic factor that I'll discuss more later. Why dendrites? They are the inputs to the synapse, or the receiving end for neuro-signaling, and the deciders when it comes to the neuron firing (send the signal on or not). After we learn something, it gets into the storage pantry (hippocampus) through long-lasting changes in the connections between neurons in a process called consolidation. We can reactivate these memories (called re-consolidation) or extinguish or get rid of them. If there is no reason for retaining the memory, or if what was learned is not needed, then why take up space in the pantry? This is joy of forgetting! I remember reading that if we remembered everything that we took in through our senses daily that we would go crazy and that this was a role for the ECS. Forgetting, or culling the hundreds or thousands of bits of information we take in that are irrelevant or inconsequential, is a normal adaptive process for survival—not necessarily a breakdown in memory.*

We will discuss memory loss that occurs in dementia or AD that is beyond the healthy forgetting.

When we take in information, neurons get excited as neurotransmitters fire across the ends of the dendrites. This changes the connection points between the neurons, and makes a memory. The more a memory is revisited or repeated, then the change in the connection (creating a new synaptic connection) gets stronger. What happens when a relay station or connection goes unused? Think of abandoned buildings and the overgrowth and decay that can occur. The brain can't afford this type of trash accumulation in order to function at its best. The brain needs a good housecleaning every night, and thanks to clock genes this occurs. This may be one reason that a good night of sleep should result in a clear mind.

Synaptic pruning is something that occurs on a large scale from early childhood into adulthood. We are born with many more neurons than we seem to need. The brain achieves its adult status, completion of prefrontal cortex development and pruning, by around age 28. Microglia, the macrophages of the brain, are intimately involved in the pruning process, where they engulf and eliminate synapses during development (called phagocytosis). Microglia have also been shown to maintain the health of synapses and to be particularly active while we sleep! Microglia and sleep are in charge of removing dead neurons from the brain, repairing and protecting the CNS, and destroying pathogens and removing misfolded proteins. We are born to forget and the memory consolidation process overrides the mechanism of forgetting, or helping us to store memories that we need.

---

* Consider reading *Forgetting: The Benefits of Not Remembering. By Scott A Small*

Dendrites

Dendrites are outgrowths that behave as antennae, to help collect signals for the neuron. They are integral to shaping the activity of neurons, mediating complex behavior and crucial for plasticity, which is a highly dynamic process. Imagine an underground root system that is branching out in every direction. In fact, this is exactly what fungal mycelium does in the soil, acting as a communication system between plants! If a dendrite makes a new connection by synapsing with a neighboring neuron, this causes the dendrite to be more likely to continue to develop. Alternatively, those without reinforcement will not make synapses and will recede.

We can have new functional dendrites in about 12 hours. The dendritic feedback signal requires 2-AG, mediated by CB1R. Dendrites that don't stay around are considered to simply recede, a tightly regulated balance between formation and elimination, necessary for healthy brain functioning. When dendrites are no longer needed for the functional circuit, or if the circuit strength is not strong enough, they gradually diminish.

Agonists at the CB2R help to skew the macrophage/microglia to a phenotype for helping with ongoing pruning of unneeded synapses. This also underscores the role of the ECS in resolving inflammation and damage in the brain.[195] In neurodegenerative diseases, the microglia will act as phagocytes, where they move toward damage site, including ischemic damage (from stroke), excitotoxic damage (can occur from glutamate), and neurodegenerative processes (such as in PD), where these monocytes of the brain engulf and eliminate neuronal debris after cell death.

Extinction of Memory

A brain structure called the amygdala, a hub for emotional processes, plays a primary role in acquiring, storing, and extinction of aversive memories. There is a process gone awry when an emotional memory that is no longer needed persists. Storing aversive memories are a necessary part of survival, but after time, when the memory is not reinforced, behavioral responses should eventually become extinct or suppressed. Animal studies have revealed that activation of the CB1R in the amygdala, another brain area rich in CB1R, is essential for extinction of fearful memories.[196] Failure to do so is a core mechanism behind PTSD symptoms.

The classic example of this type of conditioning is Pavlov's dogs (Ivan Pavlov was a researcher who studied conditioned reflexes) that were trained to connect the ringing of a bell with feeding. The dogs would begin to salivate when hearing the bell ring, anticipating food. Over time if the bell continued to ring, but no food was provided, the dog eventually stopped running to the food bowl when the bell was rung. Pavlov was the first to use the term extinction to describe this loss of memory.[197] This type of conditioning, with a lack of extinction, is the case in PTSD where there is an impairment in the ability to get rid of memories of traumatic experiences or behavioral responses to a trigger. This is evidenced by heightened arousal to a cue (such as a loud noise being perceived as gunfire) and hypervigilance to surroundings. These responses are connected to the amygdala, which is writing the code, so-to-speak, creating the association between the trigger and the response.

Mice that are deficient in CB1R, or treated with an antagonist (blocker) of the receptor, proved that endocannabinoids are allowing for extinction of aversive memory in the amygdala.[198] Deficiency in endocannabinoids has been measured in the blood of victims who met diagnostic criteria for PTSD of the 9/11 attack on the World Trade Center, compared to healthy controls.[199] 2AG was reduced while AEA, PEA, and OEA levels went up and correlated with decreased cortisol levels (reflecting the relationship between the ECS and the HPA: See Chapter 3: Relax). Inhibiting the breakdown of 2AG (MAG lipase inhibitors) is one strategy being explored. In animals, this approach seems to convert the animals from being susceptible to being resilient to a stressor.[200] Eventually, being able to easily measure the changes in the ECB levels may result in their ultility as biomarkers for stress. An early-stage experiment suggests that boosting AEA, by inhibiting its degrading enzyme (FAAH), may be a treatment approach—boosting AEA levels in the brain may help with the extinction of aversive memories.[201]

While fear should be normal, adaptive and survival-oriented, some learned behaviors can become maladaptive. Maladaptivity can include fear responses from stimuli such as sights, smells, sounds, or being in the context of a traumatic event. The coming together of all of these sensory memories and failure to extinguish associations from situations such as combat, ACEs, predator exposure, social defeat, single prolonged stress, or other trauma is what constitutes PTSD. This is a case where we forget to forget, and the ECS is central to this type of forgetting. In addition, ongoing stress can also contribute to the shrinking (atrophy) of the hippocampus leading to deficits in short-term verbal memory (cognitive problems). We will discuss this further in the section on cognitive health and AD.

Experimentally in animals, both THC and CBD have been shown to potentiate the extinction of aversive memory. Interestingly, both of these compounds likely have biphasic effects on this process, specifically a 7.5 mg dose of THC reduced negative emotional effects while a higher dose (12.5 mg) increased distress in a model of stress.[   ]

Many people may be familiar with the taking too high of a dose of THC and experiencing paranoia. This past experience is a reason some people are averse to using cannabis even for a medical purpose. Such a negative past experience is something that will cause avoiding repeating such an unpleasant experience.[202] Most CB1 agonists have been shown to have the extinction effect. While enhancing AEA levels appears to be beneficial, enhancing levels of 2AG may worsen the ability extinguish adverse memories. Genetic single nucleotide polymorphisms (SNPs) in the CB1R gene have been associated with the failure to extinguish conditioned fear in healthy people, implicating ECS genetics as causing changes that alter stress responses. Some other mutations may facilitate (FAAH SNPs) or protect against developing PTSD after traumatic experiences.

There have been few clinical studies evaluating cannabinoid compounds in patients with PTSD. Most of these have been small numbers of people who are also on other medications for PTSD. A small placebo-controlled trial of 3 cannabis potencies showed some benefit for PTSD symptoms, but not significantly better than the placebo cannabis (THC and CBD removed).[203]

Short-term improvements in quality of life were reported from a registry in the UK of medical cannabis patients who were using cannabis for PTSD.[ ] There is a need for trials in larger numbers of individuals to unveil the role of cannabis in evaluating the long-term effects on helping to resolve this deficit on fear extinction that results in debilitating symptoms for those who are susceptible.

Body/Mind Interface 5

Mental or cognitive flexibility is something that can be cultivated; if not cultivated, flexibility can be lost. An agile mind is associated with our general resilience, creativity, adaptability, and to be responsive in less regimented ways. Changing our environment, attitudes, behaviors, actions and motivations can help us to feel more optimistic, reduce fear and get out of being stuck. If you find yourself in a situation where your mind seems stuck on a thought, an outcome, or even a memory, here are some ideas of things you can do:

1. Do anything different! If you are sitting, get up and take a walk outside. Exercise and looking at something new both give you a mental boost. In the longer term, you can take a vacation or consider changing your job, rearrange your house, or change up a room. Changing the scenery can make a big difference in mental attitude.

2. Learn something new! Novelty encourages mental flexibility and also supports brain growth. Taking a language class, dance class, or learning a new musical instrument can have this effect. Simpler is trying a new recipe, listening to a variety of music, or eating at a new restaurant—all help to increase creativity and enhance problem-solving

3. If you are stuck in your ways, determine that you will be more spontaneous. Change any routine that you are in, even changing the streets you drive to go to the store. Eat dinner for breakfast. Getting out of habitual ruts will help your brain ruts to be less entrenched.

4. Question yourself by listening to your thoughts or conversations. Try to see if you are attached to any way of thinking about something or are rigid about your attitudes toward anything. Actively try out

different perspectives from those you believe in. This will make you more approachable, more positive, and less rigid in how you think.

5. Mix up what you are doing. Instead of staying focused on something for long periods of time, consider taking exercise snacks (5 minutes of vigorous activity) or do something creative for 20 minutes (like drawing, playing an instrument, dancing). If you allow your brain to un-focus and activate the DFN, you may find that you can be more creative, innovative, and satisfied with your work!

Psychedelics

A psychedelic is a drug that causes expansions of and alterations of consciousness and hallucinations; it literally means mind-manifesting. Cannabis (THC specifically) is considered to be a psychotropic drug, not a psychedelic. A psychotropic drug affects brain function leading to changes in mood, awareness, thoughts, feelings, or behaviors (caffeine, nicotine, and alcohol are included in this class of drugs).

Effects of psychedelics are well-known to occur through tryptamine compounds acting or binding to serotonin receptors (5-hydroxy tryptamine: 5HT), notably the 5HT2A receptor. Psychedelics have been used across cultures since written history began. They have been used in traditional healing practices in plant-based medicines, in Indigenous community experiences and to incite mystical experiences as a regular part of spiritual practice. They are generally considered not to lead to addiction. The cultures represented include Indigenous Americas/Turtle Island people, Indian, the Mazatec, Huichol, Shipibo, and other nations as well as the Maya, Olmec, Zapotec, and Aztec pre-Columbian societies. There was a sacred positioning of many plants in these cultures and communities. Hallucinations are not necessarily what many of these drugs do to *most* users at *ordinary* doses (dose-response effects). These plant medicines are now used in therapeutic settings with guided psychoanalysis—psychedelic therapy—to treat persons with anxiety, depression, and PTSD. As with THC, intoxicating effects are dose-related.

Interestingly, a report in 2021 in the journal *Neuron* reported that psilocybin from the mushroom *Psilocybe* induces dendritic spine growth and structural remodeling in the first 24 hours after dosing and persisted during the month following the experiment.[204] This may indicate a mushroom-based mechanism that promotes neuroplasticity. This type of plasticity aiding in the remodeling of the brain helps with depression and may be useful for other neuropsychiatric disorders such as addiction, PTSD, dementias/AD, and OCD. The ability for the brain to rewire, make new connections, and compensate for areas that are lost is essential for PD patients, pain patients, and those with autism spectrum disorder (ASD) to make new connections and naturally heal.

Psychedelics are thought to affect the integrity of the DMN, the network our brain defaults to or is active when we're not processing the outside world. The DMN is thought to be associated with memory recall about ourselves, the wandering mind, or rumination. Psychedelics may act by disconnecting the hippocampus from the DMN, which then leads to a breakdown in our attachment to our personal identity. This breakdown can be transformative for some and a crisis for others, thus the need for trained persons in guiding such an experience.

Approaches for helping people with the debilitating effects of PTSD are being considered. This includes the use of *Psilocybe* mushrooms and the recent FDA application for approval of MDMA, (commonly known as ecstasy, the recreational triptan drug) both used in a trained therapist-guided experience.[205] Both of these substances act primarily through the serotonergic system. The anesthetic ketamine (known as the recreational drug special K) is considered to be a dissociative and a hypnotic drug, acting through antagonizing the glutamate receptor NMDA. Fear extinction is dependent on the activation of this receptor together with CB1R activation.

Ketamine is being widely marketed for depression and often is given without the benefit of therapy and particularly without integration therapy (therapy over time to integrate the experience). Ketamine effects are different from other anesthetics in that eyes remain open, there are no hallucinogenic effects and it is quick acting as an antidepressant but may not have long-term results. Ketamine also acts on a pain activation network (insula-thalamus-cingulate-cortex-prefrontal cortex) and effects may be potentiated by CBD and endocannabinoids.[206, 207] It tends to allow people to access traumatic memories that can allow for gaining insight and new perspectives, provide an immediate mood boost, help to decrease defensiveness, and be a catalyst for spiritual insights, driving personal growth. There is a dire need for therapies such as these that can rapidly help people and improve long-term quality of life for this patient population, such as addressing: perpetual psychological distress, changes in cognition, distressing dreams, avoidance of situations, dissociative reactions, and mood. However, the best proven treatment is still cognitive behavioral therapy.

> **HERBAN LEGEND #6** is that cannabis or THC is a hallucinogen. While there may be dose-dependent effects that vary from person-to-person, particularly a risk of psychosis for some, this is not the drug category where cannabis fits- it is a psychoactive, or mind activating drug.

The potential for THC to be hallucinogenic for select persons is relevant considering the high potencies at which people inhale THC-based products (such as vape pens and dabbing). The supra-physiologic doses in these delivery systems allow for off-target effects of THC, including binding to and activating the 5HT2A receptor, which then *could* be pro-hallucinogenic.[208] In animals, THC was shown to sensitize this receptor, a process that could lead to the increased susceptibility of psychotic or schizophrenic-type responses in people who are susceptible (based on individual genetics combined with their environments).

When the CB1R itself interacts directly with 5HT2AR (as a heteromer),* it triggers a different signaling pathway than either receptor triggers alone. This combining of 2 proteins for signaling, heterodimerization, is a way that the body uses resources wisely. The interaction of CB1/5HT2A is thought to contribute to the memory-impairment, anxiety-reducing, and

---

* A monomer is a single unit and a heteromer is this single unit combining with another different unit.

pro-social effects of cannabis. Cannabis does share some features with psychedelic drugs, such as enhanced sensory perception, visual effects (but not seeing things that are not there as with visual hallucination), emergence of previously unrecognized emotions, abstract thought patterns, and creative thinking—all effects experienced with psychedelics at low to moderate doses.

A 65-year-old friend of mine told me yesterday that loud noises still take him directly back to his childhood, acting as a trigger for his sympathetic nervous system. His dad used to slam things down and curse when he was a boy. His behavioral response is to dissociate, or feel disconnected from himself and the world around him. This can manifest as the mind blanking out, closing the eyes or staring into space, loss of motor function, and rapid mood swings—a normal way to respond to traumatic events. This is like the passive defense mode called freezing, which is an immobility due to shutting down of the arousal system (activation of the vagus nerve).

The problem in this instance is that his dad is no longer alive and this is now a maladaptive behavioral response to a loud noise. This illustrates that, just as a group people can be exposed to the same trauma and some have PTSD and others not, individually we can have specific triggers AND we can reprogram the brain to not react to them.

Depersonalization is an effect that cannabis reportedly can cause. This is described as a dissociative symptom, where one feels to be an outsider, detached from surroundings, and is a transient situation that can be a part of the euphoric experience of cannabis and helpful experience in the face of trauma or a cause of impairment and distress that can be part of a psychotic psychiatric disorder (affecting 2% of the population worldwide). For my friend, cannabis is an herbal ally for him, helping him to be more calm, less reactive to the environment, and helps his brain consider other options.

Executive Function

Working memory is associated with the real-time processing of information, comprehension of new inputs, problem-solving, and executive function—what could be called primary memory or the things within our consciousness. It is a small amount of information used to execute tasks (following a set of instructions), contrasting with long-term memory, and helps us stay on task and manage the information we need in real time. Working memory is also important for learning and can be thought of as attention span.

Executive function (EF) is what allows for us to focus our attention, remember instructions, put things together in order, plan, stay on task, multitask, and have cognitive flexibility. Acute intoxication with THC can cause problems with multiple areas of EF and is typically limited to the few hours immediately after use, but can be longer lasting for some people and bleed into the next day. There are likely interactions occurring between the ECS and dopaminergic and GABAergic neurotransmission. AEA and 2AG appear to have opposite effects on EF in humans, as elevated levels of AEA were associated with cognitive flexibility and improved decision-making while 2AG elevation was associated with the opposite.[209] There are also biphasic effects of agonists at CB1R, showing that high dose *increased* impulsive behavior (this would cause us to deviate from tasks) while a low dose of a CB1R antagonist *reduced* impulsive responses.[210]

Actions of the ECS related to impaired EF may be explained by changes in neurotransmitter release (dopaminergic, cholinergic, GABAergic, and glutamatergic), but more likely to alteration in functional connectivity. Cannabis, particularly when under the acute intoxication phase, is likely to cause us to forget what we were doing, to be distracted, for our thoughts to become tangential or hyper-fast and connecting things we might not normally connect. On the other hand, this is an experience that recreational users interpret as being creative. Given that a host of creative people may have brain function that is similar to what occurs in schizophrenia or in the manic phase of bipolar disorder, thinking outside the box may be beneficial sometimes.[211] Results may vary, as heavy use can also be associated with adverse events such as an acute psychotic episode and for those at risk, developing chronic schizophrenia, even after stopping cannabis use.

Those who initiate use of cannabis at young ages have an earlier age of onset of schizophrenia than people who have never used drugs. The association of cannabis with schizophrenia is not something that can be ignored. In addition to dopamine signaling, interruption of the salience network may contribute to these effects.

In animals, there is clearly a dose-related role in working memory or EF, matching the concept of biphasic effects. Remember that THC is considered a partial agonist, while ECBs are full agonists at CB1R. Also, the way that THC binds the receptor is likely different from that of ECBs, as there are several chemical structures of cannabinoid compounds and they have slightly varied binding pockets in the protein structure. Binding of each structural type will orient the protein in different ways. This change in protein conformation results in what is known as biased signaling, meaning the protein structure dictates what happens next in signal transduction. This varied signaling will in turn have functional implications.

Reinforcement Learning

Release of the neuromodulator DA is critical to the control of movement, motivation, and reward. DA is the main neurotransmitter that has been intimately linked with addictive behaviors. DA is a key neurotransmitter in EF, and the DA2 receptor (D2R) is a GPCR, and is the primary target for antipsychotic drugs (risperidone, ropinirole). Dysregulation of DA signaling underpins psychosis and schizophrenia, 2 mental health conditions that have been associated with cannabis use. High levels of DA can lead to dysregulated behavior, such as mania or hypomania. Mania or manic behavior is extremely high energy levels (hyperactivity) with elevation in mood (euphoric or irritable) that feels like self-importance, getting easily distracted (flight of ideas), having a lot of new ideas and plans (sometimes bordering on delusion), disturbed illogical thinking, and the decreased need for sleep. Manic behavior is usually associated with lack of sleep, sometimes for days, while hypomania is a milder version of mania that usually lasts a few days, but may not be associated with sleeplessness. The ECS can negatively modulate the D2R. For example, in humans with schizophrenia, levels of AEA are elevated at all stages of the illness, and antipsychotic drugs may work in part to bring these levels back to homeostasis.

As humans, we often have to make decisions and sometimes our actions are based on whether or not we get any reward. This type of learning has been linked to DA neurons and what has become known as the reward pathway in the brain. The ventral tegmental area (VTA) is where DA is released, providing a feeling of pleasure. The VTA sends signals through the meso-limbic pathway which includes signals to the amygdala, the hippocampus (remember this!), nucleus accumbens (mediating motivation, particularly involving the motor system), and prefrontal cortex (attention and planning—"I'm going to do this again"). Selecting actions that provide benefit is the mark of intelligence among organisms (rats, pigeons, and primates can also do this). We experience a stimulus (such as food, sex, social interactions, and addictive drugs) that basically tell our body "this is good and I want more." Overactivation of this reward circuit can result in addictions and addictive behaviors.

THC and DA

The effects of THC on the dopamine (DA) system are considered to contribute to recreational and potentially harmful effects. Endocannabinoids are abundant in the dopaminergic pathways, where they act as a feedback system to modulate dopamine neurotransmission. Both AEA and 2AG have been shown to stimulate dopamine release in the nucleus accumbens (NAC), a key interface between motivation and action, part of the mesolimbic pathway.* Both increases and decreases in DA signaling by THC, depending on the dose, have been reported. Low dose of THC may help to increase the conversion of DA's starting molecule tyrosine, to DA, while high doses decrease this synthesis or blunt the dopaminergic system.

This is another example of biphasic effects of THC. All of the findings, taken together, suggest that THC increases the firing rates of DA neurons, and synthesis and subsequent release of DA. Does this mean that THC, by increasing DA, results in a person becoming addicted to cannabis? Not necessarily, because the THC-induced DA release is typically less than that

---

* The mesolimbic pathway is considered to be the reward system in the brain. Release of dopamine activates the salience network for incentive, and brings a sense of pleasure. Depletion of dopamine in this pathway is related to depression.

caused by other highly addictive drugs (cocaine, amphetamine). I think of highly addictive drugs releasing a flood of DA, while THC releases a trickle. However, results may vary and this is likely dependent on individual genetics. The acute DA release is likely participating in the experience of the munchies since appetite is also modulated by the DA system. Chronic use of THC may deplete DA synthesis capacity, and this is probably seen in the situation of cannabis use disorder (CUD), also associated with poor working memory and potentially depression.

As a word of caution, mutations in elements of the DA system machinery are linked to the risk for psychosis and schizophrenia, particularly in combination with high-dose THC use.[212] These effects could include hypersensitivity of D2 receptors to DA, impaired ECS regulation of DA signaling, and impairments in metabolizing DA (MAO and COMT enzyme mutations). There are still challenges in understanding all of these complex effects, particularly that of the effects of long-term THC exposure on the DA system. The adolescent brain appears to be particularly vulnerable, and given that many teens access vape pens, highly concentrated THC, and dabbing (also high THC content), this represents a dire need for education of our teens and watchfulness over the availability of these products to young people.

Functional Connectivity

Neurons do not act in isolation, but through networks or circuits, just like electrical connections in an electronic device. These are functional networks, by which the internal flow of information in the brain adapts to external inputs. Think of it like computer software that is programmed and can be updated. Functional connectivity measures connections (electrical activity or oxygen use) between different brain structures that use tracts of nerve fibers or axons (called white matter; gray matter is dense in neuronal cell bodies).

For fear-related memories, the network includes the amygdala-hippocampus-prefrontal cortex circuit (the newest part of the brain that is well developed in humans) and increased amygdala-insula-anterior cingulate nucleus circuit activity. In the case of addiction, strengthened connectivity in the mesolimbic pathway occurs. fMRI is being exploited to bring insight into this process. By studying the brain and looking at all of its connections and mapping patterns, we can further understand brain function in the setting of many diseases in the brain such as PD, AD, cardiovascular disease, drug abuse, and how cannabis impacts the brain.

Functional connectivity in the brain is altered by cannabis use both in the short term and in the long term, helping us to understand better both cognitive and behavioral changes associated with cannabis use. With chronic cannabis use, the CB1R expression diminishes but can quickly start to recover and be back to normal with 4 weeks of abstaining from use.[213-215] It appears that overall, intoxication with THC causes reductions in the mesolimbic circuit; the salience network correlates with changes in cognitive function and psychoactive effects, including psychosis. The salience (quality of being important) of an input or stimulus determines whether it is relevant for our brain to take into account. This is a key brain mechanism that facilitates learning and survival, by allowing our focus to be engaged only the most important events, given that we have limited resources for focusing. THC seems to override the salience aspect of the network by causing us to think that an insignificant event is now significant. This overriding occurred at THC doses of 10 mg, a dose that is often used as a single-dose reference in cannabis dispensaries.[216] CBD at 300 mg in this the same study of healthy subjects had opposite effects from THC. The authors do not rule out that the effects may also be attributed to increased blood flow (through dilation of blood vessels by THC).

Default Mode Network

The DMN activates when our brain is at rest, and is deactivated when we are involved in a task or goal-oriented behavior. Connectivity within this network is not present in infants or children, but begins to develop during adolescence. Dysfunction of the DMN may contribute to rumination and the self-preoccupation often observed in patients with anxiety, depression, or OCD. In this case, the mind-wandering aspect becomes consumed with negative ruminations and the prefrontal cortex is engaged and hyper-fixated on past and future evaluation of events.

Conscious activation of the DMN can be a helpful means for helping to disengage the mind from past or present negative content that can lead to emotional distress. This network is also engaged in REM sleep and may be involved in dreaming. In a study of inhaled cannabis, THC administration suggested a possible role for the DMN in executive function, by decreasing the connectivity with an area of the brain called the posterior cingulate cortex (PCC) and suggesting a role for the ECS in regulating DMN activity. THC resulted in less deactivation of the PMN (meaning that it was activated) and thereby interfered with task performance and goal-oriented behavior.[217] Regular cannabis use or overuse may cause disturbances in the DMN and negatively impact mental health. This is particularly true during adolescence, the developmental period for the DMN, reinforcing the idea that cannabis may be best for mature brains only. Mindfulness-based stress reduction training may help allow us to access and reprogram the DMN.

Women's Health

The female brain is a force to be reckoned with. Because of our monthly hormonal fluctuations, brain plasticity in women is heightened which lends us to being biodiverse creatures. Too much plasticity can be problematic, an association with some hormonally-associated monthly mood derangements (PMS and PMDD). Women have a dynamic plasticity and connectivity, driven by estrogen which is neuroexcitatory, and hyperfunctioning can therefore occur on a monthly basis. I call this experience the Jablonskis. Polish physicist Aleksander Jablonski first described how light could excite molecules, causing them to jump transiently into a higher energy state (this happens with fluorescent molecules). I think this happens when estrogen levels rise across the menstrual cycle; I experience it and most of my female patients agree. Learning to tap into, tame the Jablonskis, or harness them for creative purposes is key!

FIGURE 5.2   ADAPTED JABLONSKI DIAGRAM

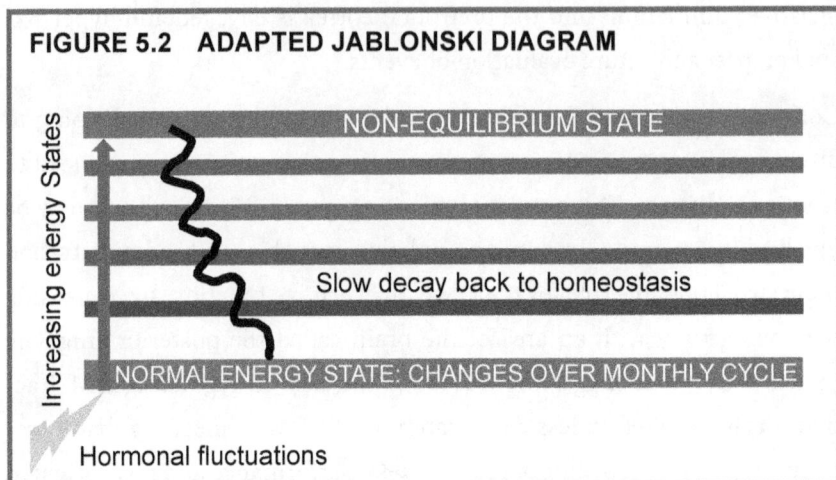

NON-EQUILIBRIUM STATE

Increasing energy States

Slow decay back to homeostasis

NORMAL ENERGY STATE: CHANGES OVER MONTHLY CYCLE

Hormonal fluctuations

Forgetting to stop being plastic (hyper-plasticity) has been associated with the type of hyperfunctioning known as neurodivergence or functioning on the autism spectrum (autism spectrum disorder: ASD). There are alterations in the ECS in ASD (low plasma anandamide) associated with mood, behavioral, and social deviations.[218] In autism, hyper-functional connectivity has been measured, particularly with the part of the brain involved in processing light.[219] Interestingly, males are more susceptible than females to develop autism; this may be partially due to a lower threshold for plasticity than females. CBD is being trialed for autism spectrum. Engaging the CB1R is a strategy for addressing this hyperfunctioning, by shifting from hyperfunctioning to inhibition. Biphasic effects of THC need to be kept in mind.

Mitochondria (Again)

The brain has more mitochondria than any other organ in our body, due to high energy demand, provided by glucose. Up to 20% of the body's energy is generated in the brain, although it is only 2% of the body's weight. Mitochondria represent 10% of our weight. This is what the enslavement of purple bacteria by an ancient ancestor of ours, the protoeukaryote, achieved.[220]

Remember that the CB1R controls our cellular respiration (cells breathe!) and energy production.[221] The CB1R is expressed on the mitochondrial membrane, which is the active site the fuel of the cell ATP, thereby the motor of our entire body. Our brain makes over 13 pounds of ATP daily! Specifically, CB1R is thought to regulate the activity of complex 1 in the process of cellular respiration. High doses of THC and 2AG have been shown to inhibit complex 1 activity, thereby reducing the generation of ATP and ROS. There are genetic mutations that lead to deficiency in complex 1 called NADH-coenzyme Q reductase deficiency. Not only is CB1R the mostly highly expressed receptor in the brain of its type, if every mitochondria has at least 1 CBR, then there are over 370 quadrillion CB1R in the body (a conservative estimate). This accounts for the majority of all proteins made by our body; This count does not include CB2R. I hope this blows your mind, as it did mine!

The ECS is the foundation of our being, the reason we can live in an oxygen-rich environment, and the sensor intended to prevent us from being killed by oxygen. The ECS regulates our oxygen consumption, literally helping us to not die from generation of excessive reactive oxygens. These are a natural byproduct of ATP production. We can be exposed to chemicals such as insecticides that inhibit complex 1 and affect our neuronal energetics. Both protecting our brain from chemicals, and supporting mitochondrial function interrupts processes that alter these energetics, and are key for optimal cognitive health.

Like the ever-changing ocean, so is the female brain. Estrogen affects brain chemistry, structure, and function, across the lifespan. This shapes our mental health, behaviors, and cognitive life. It is not surprising that as estrogen wanes, how women see the world can be altered. In archetypal psychology, the crone, which means crown, is one who intentionally honors what is of the mind. As women transition during menopause, the head, heart, and soul unite. This allows for an aerial viewpoint of life where we can finally see and call things what they are. A heightened sense of intuition, or the ability to see into our own beings, interoception develops even further. This process can be interrupted by past or current trauma, the making of bad partnerships, and by the numbing effects of certain medications that are prescribed for anxiety and depression or pain. It is never too late though to re-enter the process of becoming or embracing the wise woman archetype.

Using thoughtful approaches of psychotherapy and integrative and somatic medicines, may help to address things that have been suppressed.

Time for a Body Connection Check-in:

First place yourself on the line.

⬅——————————————————➡

++Body Awareness   **Body Detachment++**

For each question below, assess yourself on this scale: not at all, a little bit, sometimes, most of the time, all of the time.

_____ 1. I notice that my breathing becomes shallow when I am nervous.

_____ 2. I notice my emotional response to caring touch.

_____ 3. I am aware of internal sensation during sexual activity.

_____ 4. I feel separated from my physical body when I am engaged in sexual activity.

_____ 5. I notice that my body feels different after a peaceful experience.

_____ 6. When I am stressed, I notice the stress in my body.

_____ 7. When I am physically uncomfortable, I think about what might have caused the discomfort.

For each time you answered not at all, score a zero; a little bit = 1; some of the time = 2; most of the time = 3; and all of the time = 4. These questions are part of a larger survey on the Scale of Body Connection. How do you score? Statements 1, 2, 3, 5, 6, and 7 assess your body awareness so a higher score is better. Statement 4 assesses your body dissociation, so a lower score is better. The mark on the line is hopefully slowly moving toward greater body awareness as you have made your way through the book.

Alzheimer's Disease (AD)

AD is the most common neurodegenerative disease associated with aging. Since baby boomers are reaching older age, there is an upcoming epidemic of dementias and AD. Even though women tend to live longer than men, we are more likely to develop AD than men. Estrogen acting at the estrogen receptor alpha directly impacts the hippocampus and is both cognitive- and neuro-protective. This highlights estrogen and hormone therapy in the process of cognitive decline. Most of the research on hormones and the brain has focused only on women who are already postmenopausal. Estrogen promotes dendritic growth, but only in females, particularly affecting the hippocampus (the memory pantry) and cognitive function.[222] Synaptic loss is induced when estrogen levels drop after menopause, reflected by the fact that cognitive loss occurs more often in women than men.

Dementia is severe impairment and the transition to dementia is called mild cognitive impairment (MCI). MCI is a disease of midlife in women and prevention is key! Subjective cognitive impairment (SCI) occurs 10 years prior to MCI and won't be caught on any kind of cognitive testing. Our perimenopausal brain is already calling out for metabolic brain fuel.

The hippocampus is linked to memory as our memory pantry. As you age, you are likely to begin experiencing age-related memory decline. This doesn't always mean we will get dementia, but forgetfulness and difficulty with word-finding are 2 things that perimenopausal and postmenopausal women report to me. Around 20% of perimenopausal/menopausal women report changes in verbal learning, or in the ability to acquire and synthesize new information. AD is associated with the shrinking or atrophy of the hippocampus.[223] If we start early enough, we can reverse, or at the very least stabilize, this process.

AD is another neurodegenerative process associated with a proteinopathy,* in this case beta-amyloid plaque (a-beta) and tangles that are made of tau proteins. The normal role of the a-beta protein is to stabilize the cell

---

* Proteinopathies are a class of disease where misfolded proteins lose their normal function, due to the change in shape, and become toxic to organs, tissues, and cells. They can also stick together and make clumps or tangles.

membrane of the neuron. In AD, the disruption leads to loss of synapses, neurons, and activation of microglial cells or neuroinflammation. The onset of this type of dementia is usually after age 60 (considered late onset) and makes up 95% of all AD diagnoses. It is typically a rapid and progressive disease characterized by decline in memory, executive function (EF), language, and motor skills, but can also include behavioral and psychological changes. It is a multicausal process than can be exacerbated by leaky gut syndrome, oxidative damage, chronic diseases (inflammation), mycotoxins, high blood sugar, vascular problems, trauma, hormonal, lifestyle patterns, and trophic factors.

There is also a link to a genetic inheritance for AD, that of the APOE4 gene. This gene that encodes for an apolipoprotein,* and carrying even 1 copy of this gene is a risk factor for developing dementia, including AD. This protein helps to carry cholesterol and other fatty acids in the bloodstream and the APOE4 mutation is associated with disruption of lipid metabolism in the brain. In cell cultures, the essential nutrient choline, needed for the synthesis of phospholipids (which make up our cellular membranes), provided benefits to this disrupted lipid metabolism.[224]

The CB1R expression has not been shown to change in the AD brain, based on tissue analysis from both humans and animal studies, but CB2R expression in microglia is overexpressed within the plaque. CB1R-expressing neurons, however, have been shown to be reduced in the areas around these microglia. AEA and CBD have both been shown to inhibit neurotoxicity associated with plaque and 2AG is also likely neuroprotective. In 2016, a group of researchers at the Salk Institute in California reported some preliminary evidence that cannabinoids may promote the removal of a-beta. [225] In this paper THC was said to be "protective, removes intra-neuronal a-beta and completely eliminates the elevated eicosanoid production" in the cells. There are no drugs on the market that have this mechanism. Meanwhile, the ability to remove this accumulation of protein is the primary strategy of drugs being developed for AD. The a-beta is promoting

---

* Apolipoproteins are proteins that bind lipids so that they can be carried around in the bloodstream.

production of pro-inflammatory lipids, illustrating a role for supplementation of omega-3 fatty acids. The data strongly suggest that early intervention to reduce the protein toxicity is imperative to reduce AD progression and initiation.

The ECS plays a role in monitoring for misfolding of proteins. This is due to the CB2 receptor being found on another organelle inside the cell, the endoplasmic reticulum, where proteins go for folding and processing. Here the CB2R acts as a sensor for a different kind of stress, more mechanical in nature. The precise role of the ECS here is still a part of the mystery of the ECS. 2AG acting at CB2R at the endoplasmic reticulum is in charge of cell fate: Will the cell live or die? It turns out that the mineral zinc is needed to help proteins not misfold. Our ECS monitors when the cell forgets to fold the protein correctly.

In women with the APOE4 genetic risk factor, the first potential plaques are starting to form during perimenopause, when estrogen starts to fluctuate. Menopause is a time in life when we could be likened to a solar collector, subject to clouds impeding our energy flow. Because of estrogen's wide influence, replacement of estrogen began to be a therapy in the 1960s, when menopause was pegged to be a "disease," hormone deficiency syndrome. This syndrome is associated with hot flashes, onset of cardiovascular disease, osteoporosis, and AD.

A man (ironically) wrote the book *Feminine Forever*. American gynecologist Robert A. Wilson claimed that estrogen would preserve femininity (whatever that is). In his opinion, femininity was equivalent to sexuality and the "physical social and psychological fulfillment" that was dependent on a woman's ability to attract and keep a suitable mate (or holding his interest)! He likened this state of feminine deficiency to decay and as being a horror.[226]

In 1975, studies of estrogen replacement therapy (ERT, which Dr. Wilson espoused in his book) had already been linked to endometrial cancer, increased risk of stroke, and of developing breast cancer. Further studies of ERT revealed that estrogen should not be given unopposed by progesterone, and hormone replacement therapy (HRT) could thus be promoting women to be healthy forever. This HRT approach of combining estrogen and progesterone reduced the risk of endometrial cancer.[227] It has also been shown to prevent osteoporosis and when given in an optimal time window (soon after or <10 years of menopause) may help to prevent cardiovascular disease.[228] For women at risk of AD (carrying the APOE4 gene), introduction of hormone replacement was shown to be associated with some protective effects highlighting the neurophysiological benefits of estrogen, but clinical trials have been conflicting.[229] It may be that the benefit is only for women who also experience hot flashes, since one small study showed that improvement in hot flashes was associated with improvement in cognitive function.

Women's heart health is known to be superior to men's until we hit menopause, at which point our risk for cardiovascular disease can quickly skyrocket—meeting that of men of similar age. An observational study of HRT in 1991 suggested a 50% decrease in the risk of heart disease. An advisory committee to the FDA in the same year suggested that all women were candidates for HRT; however, the trial actually found that there was a small increased risk of cardiac events (29%) and stroke (41%). These risks are only when HRT is given to women *after* the 10-year menopause window. No studies have yet followed women who started HRT in their 40s or 50s.

Estrogen acts positively on cell proliferation through insulin growth factor 1 (IGF1) and also regulates the sensitivity of cells to insulin. Insulin, a hormone made in the pancreas, is the key allowing for glucose to enter cells. Avoiding estrogen exposure is a means to reduce breast cancer risk, but being estrogen deficient throws women into metabolic crisis.

With glucose having a difficult time entering cells, levels are elevated in the blood. Glucose is stored in fat tissues, thus the expanding midline in midlife. Higher blood glucose leads to development of cardiovascular disease or diabetes. It also means that less glucose gets into our muscles so we can have muscle loss, leading to frailty. What is the highest glucose user in our body? The brain. IR affects our cognitive function—like diabetes of the brain. Exercise is the best way to improve insulin sensitivity; some supplements such as cinnamon and berberine can be effective, too.

Keep in mind that HRT is a cocktail of synthetic compounds not identical to those made by our body. How else could a pharmaceutical industry profit as they cannot patent natural products? To date there are no large-scale trials of bioidentical hormone replacement, but there has been an indictment of them by doctors and pharmaceutical companies that influence the FDA. Millions of women use bioidenticals and while they have never been compared to HRT, they are more amenable to being used in customized doses, an excellent idea, as this is precision medicine!

Case in Point

Someone I am very close gave me permission to share her story. I met her when she was 2 years old and I was 5, and then her family moved away. Our lives intersected again when I was a young mother and she had married a friend of my then husband, a huge surprise to us both. We quickly became very close, closer than sisters. The man she married was a Vietnam veteran and we experienced together a tragedy and tremendous trauma when, estranged from him, he shot and killed a male acquaintance of hers on her back porch. She and her children were catastrophically affected, but this was during a time when after-care for PTSD experiences were barely available.

Trauma was not a novel experience for her, as she also experienced childhood trauma, scoring 6/10 on the ACEs questionnaire. Further, she experienced the death of a beloved a few years ago in a car accident. Two years ago, she learned that she had very high cholesterol, something shared with her mom and dad. She also developed some rheumatoid arthritis, very debilitating for her as someone who loves to garden, cook and work with her hands.

Around the time that her beloved was killed, she was out on a walk and experienced symptoms like a heart attack: sudden chest pain, shortness of breath, feeling weak almost to the point of fainting. Later we learned there was no evidence of a cardiovascular blockage to the heart itself but that she likely experienced broken heart syndrome. This syndrome is when the heart muscle itself is severely affected by a toxic stressor and can produce symptoms identical to a heart attack. More recently on a stressful trip back to the US, she was experiencing severe headaches and not feeling well at all. She was stressed, dehydrated, had been partying and went to bed very late and called me unable to function. Some follow-up lab work revealed that her kidneys were stressed and that she probably had experienced a hypertensive crisis- a sudden, severe increase in blood pressure. Symptoms of this include anxiety, vision changes, confusion, chest pain, shortness of breath and severe headache.

She is now 56 years old and is living a beautiful and restorative life in another country. What her story can illustrate are the combined effects of genetics and environment on health. Revisiting the introduction to this book that detailed the broad systemic effects of trauma, she has experienced 5 of the major areas of impact: cardiovascular, mental health, immune system, endocrine system and neurological. As one of the humans who I have been associated with on the planet for the longest continual period of time, and who is very precious and necessary for me, I want to keep her around!

This is why I'm so happy that she is living a life authentic to herself, in an environment where she can nurture and nourish her being! She can bring all of the elements of toning the ECS to life. She is eating fresh anti-inflammatory foods, engaging in ritual and healing ceremonies, engaging with nature daily, using natural botanical remedies to address her health issues (using pharmaceutical intervention when necessary), dancing, dreaming, hiking, swimming, getting bodywork. Most importantly, she is striving to live a stress-free life, focused only on her interests and daily activities around her coffee farm. These lifestyle modifications and her exquisite care of the ECS will hopefully keep her around for a long time. Long enough for me to go join her in retirement in a beautiful place, I hope!

Cannabis and Heart Health

There is some information suggesting that cannabis is detrimental for cardiovascular health. Some of this information is by way of an association, wherein people with cardiovascular disease report using cannabis.[230] A recent analysis of data from almost 10,000 adults showed that people who reported a history of at least monthly cannabis use had hypertension. Monthly cannabis use was not associated with any increase in blood pressure.[231] By general consensus, THC and ECBs act on smooth muscles cells and the endothelial cells produce relaxation of the blood vessels partially due to the induction of a nitric oxide synthase.[232] CBD was also shown to reduce blood pressure in a clinical trial at doses from 225–450 milligrams, 3 times per day, for 5 weeks.[233]

Some people may have cardiovascular symptoms resulting from a rapid vasodilation that can occur after inhalation of cannabis. These symptoms can include palpitations, chest pain, and syncope (a fainting spell when enough blood can't make it to the brain resulting from low blood pressure (hypotension).[234] There is no conclusive data indicating that cannabis use is detrimental to heart health; however, the high potencies available in vape pens may change the data on this topic moving forward. Smoking cannabis or vaping high potency cannabis may also have some of the same health effects of smoking tobacco, notably effects of smoke and increased risk of developing blood clots due to endothelial dysfunction.

Women's Brains

Perimenopause is a transitional time that likely sets the stage for brain health post-menopause. A shift in the thinking about menopause includes that of neurological causes, not driven by the reproductive organs or the ovary. Estrogen stimulates glucose uptake in the brain and estrogen loss can wreak havoc on cognitive function causing brain fog during perimenopause. Perimenopause is a key time to start to intervene to reduce our risk of stroke and AD.

With normal aging, CB1R expression starts to decrease in the brain. This may be one reason why older people tend to tolerate lower doses of THC better. Targeting the ECS is a means to treat AD, by studying effects of *Cannabis* on cognitive function or disease progression in humans with AD is limited. One case report and 1 pilot study indicate there may be some efficacy in treating associated behavioral disturbances with THC. The neuropsychiatric symptoms are the most difficult to treat and commonly psychotropic drugs are used: antipsychotics, benzodiazepines, antidepressants, and antiepileptic drugs. These are off-label uses, but are either only good in the short term or ineffective.[235] Two studies have shown that THC may be effective for helping people with dementia to eat, but adverse events in older persons have to be closely watched for.

The effects of THC on healthy aging in general are likely dose-dependent, with low dose being the goal. In a study of mice, young vs. old, extremely low doses of THC improved cognition in the old mice, effects that lasted 7 weeks. These doses would be sub-intoxicating doses, suggestive of 1 mg of THC or less in a human (200–500 micrograms in a 150-pound human). Another study in mice had similar results and added that they measured epigenetic effects on proteins at the synapse of the hippocampus. The researchers showed that in the THC-treated, older mice hippocampal gene transcription was restored to that of untreated, younger mice DNA.[236] This again suggests that microdosing of THC would be the equivalent in humans, and could be a strategy for treating age-related cognitive impairments.

One way that THC has shown to do this is by increasing the level of an enzyme, sirtuin1 (S1), that is involved in hippocampal neuroplasticity and also neuroprotection.[237] S1 helps the inside of the cell to clean house by autophagy. In autophagy, sensors that are monitoring for breakdown products include mTOR and S1 pathways. S1 is also relaying information that will result in gene expression changes, DNA repair, and stress responders—how the cell survives!*

CBD has also been shown to activate S1, as has THC in sepsis.[238, 239] This evidence illustrates that deep into the heart of the cell, the nucleus,

---

* A process by which a cell breaks down and destroys old, damaged, or abnormal proteins and other substances in its cytoplasm (the fluid inside a cell). The breakdown products are then recycled for important cell functions, especially during periods of stress or starvation. Once cancer has formed, autophagy may protect the cancer cells by providing extra nutrients to them or by keeping anti-cancer drugs or other substances from destroying them. Autophagy may also affect the body's immune response against viruses, bacteria, and cancer cells.

plant-based cannabinoids augment the role of the ECS and thereby have effects on our survival and perhaps longevity. Cannabinoids can be neuroprotective, mitigating AD symptoms by promoting neuronal survival, preventing oxidation and inflammation, regulating calcium hemostasis, and inhibiting glutamate neurotoxicity. Phyto-cannabinoids hold promise of helping to clear plaques that would improve memory, cognitive, and behavior in people with AD.

Neurotrophins

The brain remodels as a result of diminishing estrogen. Estrogen is known to act in concert with BDNF, a neurotrophin,* a modulator of plasticity, and is required for upregulating BDNF in adults. BDNF is one of the most prominently studied biological molecules in psychiatry for roles in stress, PTSD, and psychiatric disorders.[240] Neurotrophins (growth factors for nerves) are a good idea for aging! BDNF signaling converges with that of estrogen signaling, with effects on survival, plasticity, learning, and growth. In the face of declining estrogen, we can still boost BDNF and preserve some signaling pathways important to cognitive health. BDNF soars during ovulation. Erinacine A, found in the *Hericium erinaceus* or Lion's mane mushroom acts similarly to BDNF by activating a receptor that induces NGF, the first discovered biologic neurotrophin, made in high amounts in the hippocampus. It is pivotal for the function of and survival of cholinergic neurons and has implications for diabetes, neuropathy, and PD.

Modifiable Risk Factors

Remember acetylcholine? Inhibiting the breakdown of this neurotransmitter is one of the primary treatment approaches for AD with drugs such as donepezil, Aracept and Exelon. The loss of acetylcholine function is the reason we want to try to avoid all drugs that block the receptors for acetylcholine, such as benzodiazepines. Diazepam, commonly prescribed for sleep, impairs dendritic spine plasticity, and causes cognitive impairment in mice.[241]

---

* A neurotropin is a substance involved in the develmenopt and maintenance of neurons, modulating plasticity.

We already knew that these drugs do this to people, and now we have a mechanism. While sleep disorders increase our susceptibility to dementia, taking diazepam or Benadryl does the same; the cure is also the poison! If you are on any anticholinergics, stop now as this is a modifiable risk factor for dizziness, confusion, falls, cognitive decline, and dementia!*

Another consideration is dietary intake of a nutrient called choline, which our body does not manufacture. This is another modifiable risk factor, as supplementing the vitamin B-like nutrient can attenuate microglial activation, support synthesis of acetylcholine, improve motor function, and improve insulin sensitivity and mitochondrial function.[242]

Nutritionally, the effects of a standard American diet, in particular ultra-processed foods (UPF), promote mitochondrial failure due to reactive species damage and lowering the brain's energy capacity. UPF consumption has also been shown to be linked to an increased mortality for overall and certain site-specific cancers, especially ovarian cancer in women. A hormesis lifestyle is in order where we are enhancing biogenesis by removing these toxic exposures, maximizing antioxidant potential, improving blood flow, reducing how much sugar is in our blood, and avoiding toxins such as alcohol and tobacco, among many other toxins in our environments. We can enhance biogenesis, dendritic spine growth, and synaptoplastics (building synapses) and likely turn subjective cognitive dysfunction around in half of a year. Metabolic approaches are also in order so consideration of caloric restricting, intermittent fasting (IF) and timed eating are other approaches for cognitive health. IF is a safe way to induce autophagy and promote the body's natural lysosomal action that can remove, detoxify and recycle cells that are dying. By. using nutritional tools, changing habits, and modifying risk factors hopefully fewer women will convert from cognitive impairment to dementia to AD.

Stroke

A stroke is when the blood supply to the brain is transiently interrupted or reduced, leading to lack of oxygen and nutrients getting to the brain tissue

---

* There is an online calculator where you can look at the burden of medications on cholinergic functioning: https://www.acbcalc.com/

supplied by the blood vessel that has been blocked. This results in damage from either a blood clot or a narrowing of an artery causing blockage. Stroke is the fifth leading cause of death for women and 20% of women will experience stroke. This is devastating information, given that 90% of strokes are preventable.

Lifetime estrogen exposure (total length of time we are estrogen exposed) is linked to a woman's risk for stroke; more estrogen is better for protection of the brain.[243] This lifetime exposure benefit appears to last beyond menopause, after estrogen drops. Risks for stroke include high blood pressure, diabetes, smoking, high LDL cholesterol, obesity, and family history of stroke (genetics). Race is another factor as stroke occurs more often in African American, Alaska Native, American Indian, and Hispanic adults than in white adults. Other things we can control that affect risk are stress levels and associated anxiety and depression, sleep apnea, migraine headaches, lack of regular physical activity, and drinking alcohol.

The ECS is considered to be a great target for stroke prevention due to the effects of modulating this system on the tone of our blood vessels, on inflammation, and on our metabolic balance—all factors associated with stroke risk. Hypertension is probably the most important risk factor that we can address to help reduce stroke risk. The CB1 receptor expression on cells lining the blood vessels, as well as on the smooth muscle tissue surrounding the blood vessels, regulates contraction and dilation of blood vessel. We need our vessels to stay flexible across our lifespan.

A key molecule involved in dilation of vessels (constriction is what leads to high blood pressure) is nitric oxide, which drives this plasticity of the arteries (that carry blood to the tissues). This molecule is at the beginning of the clotting cascade, so could be preventive against clot formation. It blocks the platelets from being able to discharge their contents that allow them to aggregate. Too much aggregation leads to a clot. Blood hemostasis stops the flow of blood as needed when we are actively bleeding, but when the platelets forget that they can relax; they become hypervigilant to aggregate.

THC binding to CB1R is associated with the transient drop in blood pressure that occurs acutely after inhaling cannabis. (See Box 5.1) Our endocannabinoids binding the receptor perform this same service for us on a daily basis. Binding of CB1R leads to a release in nitric oxide and also upregulation of the enzyme making it in the blood vessels (iNOS).[244] There have been negative reports about cardiovascular effects of smoking (burning) cannabis on developing a thromboembolism (blood clot outside of the brain). This risk may also be elevated in persons using highly concentrated THC extracts such as dabbing and vape pens, or due to excipients and impurities that may be added to them. High dose of THC pay potentiate platelet activation while other results suggest that lower doses may inhibit thrombin from inducing clot formation.[245] Cannabidiol may be another stroke neuroprotectant by helping to reduce damage after a stroke.

I typically recommend CBD for any type of brain injury, neuroinflammatory or neurodegenerative condition as a neuroprotectant and to help with brain repair.[246] There is an ongoing clinical trial to look at effects of CBD on a specific type of stroke risk.[247-249] CB1R increases after stroke and accessing this receptor with low-dose THC could promote the neuroprotective effects as well as activate CB2R to tone inflammatory pathways after stroke.[250] Cannabinoids have been named by the federal government in a patent as neuroprotectants, a claim that no drug has ever gained FDA approval for.

It's clear that 1) we can significantly modify our risk for stroke and 2) that the ECS has a clear role in the pathophysiology of stroke. Toning the endocannabinoid system, especially during the sensitive postmenopausal time of life, is important, but prevention is key! Upregulating CB2R by using dietary cannabinoids will enhance anti-inflammatory effects of signaling through this receptor.

Menstrual and Pelvic Pain

The uterus is a hollow muscular organ that sits in our pelvic girdle, sandwiched by the bladder and the rectum. The mouth of the uterus, the cervix, is the gate by which our monthly fluids flow out through the vagina. There are 3 layers of muscle, an intermediate layer highly enriched with blood vessels that is sandwiched by 2 layers of smooth muscle. The myometrium has the most contractility, and can vary over the course of our menstrual cycle. CB1R is highly expressed in the uterus, although expression varies across the menstrual cycle. Progesterone in the secretory phase of the moon cycle upregulates CBR. Women with period pain also have elevated levels of AEA.[251] The endometrium is the inner layer of cells lining the womb which rapidly proliferates in response to estrogen during the proliferative phase of the moon cycle.

BOX 5.1   CANNABIS POTENTIAL ACUTE SIDE EFFECTS

1. Interference with your balance
2. Eye irritation (dryness)
3. Throat irritation (dryness or cough)
4. Increased heart rate (usually transient)
5. Possible low blood pressure (usually transient)
6. Reversible problems with your appetite (typically increase in appetite)
7. Feeling tired or slowed down (only an short-term effect)

Less Likely Cannabis Side Effects

8. Some change in your mood (good or bad)
9. Loss of memory (this is usually short lasting and not a long-term effect)
10. Decreased ability to concentrate or think properly (this is usually short lasting and not a long-term effect)

Rare but Serious Cannabis Side Effects

11. Dizziness
12. Head and chest pressure
13. Disorientation
14. Agitation
15. Combativeness
16. Incoherence
17. Visual hallucinations
18. Paranoia

The nerves supplying the organs inside the pelvis get their supply from our 11–12 thoracic nerve, getting autonomic, sympathetic (sacral nerves 2–4) and parasympathetic signals. Interestingly, the uterus and cervix are not sensitive to either burning or cutting, but they are both sensitive to stretch (which happens during pregnancy and birth). Gynecologic problems associated with the uterus include fibroids (usually benign), infections, adhesions, polyps (usually asymptomatic), adeno- and endometriosis, and cancer. We already discussed unopposed estrogen and there are other sources of xenoestrogens that act as endocrine disruptors.

One of the most common moon-time complaints is menstrual cramps or period pain. This is a situation where an herbal uterine tonic such as *Angelica sinensis* (dong qui) and *Rubus idaeus* (red raspberry) are always included in treatment. This is specifically for normalizing muscle function and to produce coordinated contractions.

For pain, antispasmodic herbs are helpful such as *Paeonia lactiflora* (Chinese peonie) with *Glycyrrhiza glabra* (licorice) or *Caulophyllum thalictroides* (blue cohosh). A suppository of cannabis, containing THC and used either vaginally or rectally, can help with the pain itself. Starting with a suppository (25–50 mg THC) a few days prior to the moon time is what was recommended in the late 1800s.[252] There is a story that Queen Victoria used it for her monthly discomforts and moon-time muscle spasms, or dysmenorrhea.[253]

If there is an inflammatory component to the pain, diet and exercise are the first-line approach. If the pain is primarily visceral or due to pain generation at the level of the nervous system, using nervine herbs and reducing stress are essential elements. Cannabis is the most potent anodyne or analgesic herb and women have used this herb long before men recommended it in their textbooks. *Piscidia erythrina* (Jamaican dogwood) and *Corydalis* can help with pain, but treating the underlying cause is essential. IBS, endometriosis, constipation, liver stagnation, and nutrition, including iron deficiency, need to be addressed.

Beyond moon time, chronic pelvic pain can include pain during intercourse, when sitting for a long time, standing a long time, or even when using the toilet. Chronic pelvic pain can be debilitating for both men and women, and up to 20% women are affected. It is considered to be a form of complex regional pain syndrome, where part of the problem is a low threshold for pain.

Sometimes it is a form of visceral neuropathy, which could be addressed by cannabis, but all other causes need to be ruled out.[254] In neuropathic pain, the most effective means for pain control is by inhalation of the cannabis, due to the rapid uptake and distribution to the brain, but suppositories work for some people (men or women, particularly if back pain is associated with the pelvic pain).

Most of the time, cannabis can be used along with other prescribed therapies and/or to help wean off other pain medications. Women who use cannabis to help with pelvic pain reported improvements in libido, cramping, muscle spasms, sleep disturbances, anxiety, irritability, and depression.[255] Sometimes problems with the bladder can be causing pelvic pain and so attention to that organ is also in order. Cannabis has been recognized as a diuretic and vasodilator, so can promote urine flow. Pelvic physical therapy is rehabilitative and can help to improve dysfunction in the pelvic floor that can contribute to pain.

Migraine

There is evidence supporting the role of the ECS in migraine through activation of CB1R.[256] This activation has been shown to modulate the activity of the trigeminovascular system (TVS), a key player in migraine. [257-260] There is also a hypothesis that low functioning of the ECS may be associated with chronic migraine.[261] In one study, AEA levels in CSF were found to be significantly less in patients with chronic migraine compared to healthy people. This may be indicative of a failure of the ECS to inhibit activation of the TVS.[262] Mechanisms of ECS modulation in migraine may include roles in the perception and transmission of pain, regulation of neurotransmitter release (including inhibiting serotonin signaling and thereby reducing pain, aura, and nausea/vomiting), tone of blood vessels, and reduction in inflammation.

Sir William Osler, considered by many the father of modern medicine, wrote in his 1916 textbook that cannabis was "probably the most satisfactory remedy" for migraine.[263] However, over 100 years later, the clinical evidence supporting the use of cannabis for migraine is still largely anecdotal. A case series from 1974 reported inhaled cannabis provided benefit for 3 patients suffering from headache and migraine.[264] More recently, a cross-sectional survey of medical cannabis users in Israel reported that among 145 respondents who received a medical cannabis authorization and self-treated with cannabis, 61% reported a ≥50% reduction in monthly migraine attacks and were categorized as responders while 31% reported <50% reduction and were categorized as non-responders.[265] The results pointed to a long-term reduction in migraine frequency, and reduced medication intake.

A retrospective chart review from 2 cannabis specialty clinics in Colorado found that 121 patients reported reduced frequency of migraine over time. The review reported a reduction in use of other pharmaceutical medications, lower scores on the Migraine Disability Assessment, and a decrease in migraine frequency from 10.4 to 4.6 episodes per month ($p<0.0001$).[266] Most participants used a combination of inhaled and oral forms daily, with inhalation used for acute treatment.

An observational study of cannabis use for migraine or headache conducted using data collected using the Releaf smartphone application reported that people with migraine using inhaled cannabis flower had mean headache pain benefit of -3.3 points on a 0–10 scale within 2 hours of administration.[267] The only randomized controlled trial (RCT) of cannabis for headache to date studied oral nabilone (synthetic D9-tetrahydrocannabinol: THC) versus ibuprofen for medication overuse headache.[268]

I am involved with a pain/migraine neurology specialist at UCSD in conducting the first clinical trial of inhaled cannabis for acute migraine. Each participant treated 4 separate migraine attacks with either placebo cannabis, low-dose THC, equal amounts of THC and CBD, or high CBD cannabis. THC/CBD mix was superior to placebo at achieving pain relief at 2 hours and also for freedom from the most bothersome migraine symptom (these results are in the process of publication).

In other news, cluster headache, an uncommon form of headache that is located on one side of the head may be responsive to *Psilocybe* according to a microdosing study. HA subjects took 0.143 mg/kg pulsed for 3 doses, each 5 days apart.[269] Those with chronic attacks had a reduced incidence in the frequency of headaches and there were no serious adverse events. This was considered to be a small, exploratory study and provided evidence that this therapy approach should be further investigated.

Breast Cancer

Many women ask their doctors about their individual breast cancer (BC) risk, as 1 out of 8 women will have a diagnosis (1 in 4 for any type of cancer). Women of all ages have an increased risk of BC after about 5 years of taking hormone replacement. While use of HRT overall has been associated with increased BC risk, it may be mostly associated with synthetic progesterone, or progestins.[270]

There is conflicting information about the role of the ECS in development of BC. Some studies suggest an overactivated ECS may be cancer-promoting while others report that ECS activation could reduce tumor growth.[271, 272] Because potential antitumor actions of cannabinoids have been reported, BC is another instance where someone may be tempted to try to treat BC using cannabis. Be aware that there are several types of BC and, overall, BC has become pretty treatable, especially when caught early. The applications for cannabis for helping during cancer treatment have been addressed by the National Cancer Institute and these include potential benefits for pain including chemotherapy-induced neuropathy, anorexia, nausea, and vomiting associated with chemotherapy, sleep, anxiety, and general quality of life.[273]

Estrogen or estradiol is the mother compound in our body metabolized (to estriol and estrone and others) through several enzyme pathways. Some of these pathways result in estrogen metabolite that is harmful to our DNA. The compound found in broccoli and other members of that family of vegetables, DIM, can help to shift estrogen metabolism to the less harmful metabolite (2-hydroxy to 4-hydroxy ratios).[274] Again, overall estrogen exposure across the lifespan is considered to be a risk factor. Other estrogen exposures are those to exogenous or xenoestrogens (see Chapter 4: Protect re endocrine disruptors)* and evaluating risk should include these compounds. It is possible to have your metabolites tested to find out how you are metabolizing estrogen.

Osteoporosis

Who would have thought that bone has cannabinoid receptors? I did not at first because bone is just this hard structural material, right? It turns out that bone is highly plastic or experiences ongoing bone remodeling. Returning to a common theme, macrophage-like cells in bone are at the heart of this plasticity. There are 2 types: osteoblasts that build bone and osteoclasts that degrade bone. These cells are equipped with the ECS, express CB2R that when activated induces bone formation by osteoblasts, and controls the crosstalk between blasts and osteoclasts. In fact, mutations in the CB2 gene may be a risk factor for the development of osteoporosis.[275] Again we see the ECS involved in tissue homeostasis, relevant in the scenario of aging, where bones forget to keep remodeling. Activity is a primary stimulus for this remodeling, another reason that staying active is so important to aging.

At the heart of bone is collagen, and collagen is a structural material throughout our tissues that is upregulated by estrogen. (Even when used topically, estrogen cream or suppositories can help with vaginal pain after menopause.) HRT has been shown to reduce the risk of fracture in post-menopausal women.[276] Collagen content drops by as much as 2% each year after menopause and includes loss of collagen in bones.**

Bone mineral density (BMD) is the measurement for risk of osteopenia (early stage of loss of BMD) and osteoporosis (strength of bone is diminished and at risk for fracture). Aging is associated with risk of bone fracture, as bone quality or the intrinsic toughness of the bone affects its plasticity, causing bone to be more likely to develop microcracks and fractures.

---

* A website to investigate your body products is https://www.ewg.org/skindeep/.

** Natural aging includes the development of fine wrinkles, skin becoming more lax, and in some cases sagging. Add the effects of sun damage and add coarse wrinkles, dryness, and lots of pigmentation, or spots.

Staying active, specifically with balance exercises (walking, dancing, stair-climbing, jogging, tai chi, yoga) and resistance exercise (weight training, swimming, cycling) can increase bone mass. Taking part in each type of exercise is important for reducing your risk of osteoporosis.

In animals, CBD was shown to upregulate a factor that helps collagen to cross-link and thereby help improve healing of fracture.[277, 278] It's not yet known if this same effect could help in humans, but is being tested for dogs. In cell cultures, CBD was shown to induce osteoblasts, an application that could help in bone regeneration. While we know that bone biology includes the ECS, the precise way to tap into this system for promoting bone health and doses of cannabinoids that might do this are unknown. Essential nutrients that are key in the support of bone health are vitamin D, vitamin K, magnesium, calcium, phosphorus, potassium, boron, zinc, manganese, and copper.

Neurological Disorders

The ECS has a range of regulatory functions in the central nervous system, and also neuroregulatory and neuroprotective roles important for brain health. As previously discussed, the ECS helps with neuronal survival, modulating immune responses (such as microglial activation), plays a role in triggering autophagy or removing damage, and is involved in antioxidant and anti-inflammatory responses. The primary role of the ECS in cellular-level homeostasis allows for stressed cells to either survive or commit cell suicide. This is an important process in neurons because damage to this cell population is not reversible. Neurological damage typically is associated with motor, cognitive, and sensory disability. CB receptors actions of being anti-inflammatory, antioxidant, anti-emetic, antiepileptic, antipsychotic, and neuroprotective lend the ECS as a promising target for neurological diseases, most of which do not hold hope for cures.

There is evidence in many neurological diseases of alterations in ECS signalling and function, and until there are drugs available that target specific elements of the ECS, phyto-cannabinoids are the only option to palliate symptoms. It is the intersection of the nervous system and immune system where cannabinoids really shine, offering hope for neuroinflammatory and neurodegenerative disorders. In fact, immune cells have been said to be mirrors of the brain. The microglia listen in to the neurons and then communicate with the body through chemical signalling then relay this through the CSF/glymphatic system to the rest of the immune system. The brain and immune system have a lot in common as well (see Box 5.3)!

BOX 5.3 SIMILARITIES BETWEEN THE NERVOUS AND IMMUNE SYSTEMS

- Are sensitive to influences from the environment
- Are prone to placebo effects and can be conditions
- Have innate and acquired responses, based on exposures
- Have both short- and long-term memories
- Highly variable across individuals and can discriminate between self and non-self
- Have the potential to become highly reactive, even to something that is not really a threat
- Can cause internal disorders such as autoimmunity or schizophrenia
- Are the products of evolution

Pain

What is pain? Pain is a perception. Incoming messages from our senses or sensory nerves (feeling) are processed in the brain-known as nociception, or the processing of noxious stimulus. Nociception (perceiving pain) results due to a complex of sensory, cognitive, and emotional factors, or a shitstorm of signals. Any chronic pain, defined as an unpleasant sensory and emotional experience associated with actual or potential tissue damage, lasting over 3–6 months is common, especially in older adults. The body somehow forgets to turn off the pain-signaling system.

Pain and chronic pain affect the quality of life of over 100 million Americans and 100 billion worldwide. The costs of inadequate pain therapy in the US have been estimated at $635 billion annually, while loss of quality of life is priceless. Chronic pain, one of the most common reasons adults seek medical care, has been linked to restrictions in mobility and daily activities, dependence on opioids, anxiety, depression, sleep deprivation, and reduced quality of life.

The initiation of pain is induced by a bodily experience, such as an injury or damage to tissue (heat, cold, chemical) or nerves (neuropathic pain), whereby our immune system, nervous system, and ECS are activated. This occurs through ion channels using sodium, chloride, and calcium as the ions. The pain experience is also modulated by a constellation of factors such as mood, meaning, and cognitive states (expectations)—there is a dynamic interaction between all of these processes. Our previous experience can condition us and dramatically either worsen pain or help to resolve it.

Pain Transmission

There is a demonstrated role of the ECS in the regulation of pain transmission, and a preponderance of preclinical research showing that exogenous cannabinoids can modulate both the perception of pain and pathology in our body. Pain processing occurs within the peripheral and central nervous systems, and cannabinoid receptors are located all along this pathway, from the tips of primary sensory afferents (carrying the signal to the brain) to the dorsal root ganglia (a relay station on the way to the brain), to the thalamus, and eventually somatosensory cortex (processing of touch, temperature, and pain). Homeostasis of pain signaling should be restored through healing of tissue injury, but sometimes this process goes awry. Termination of the acute (short-term) phase of pain, but sometimes the repetitive pain signaling leads to changes in protein expression and pain mediators resulting in a process called wind-up. The neuronal modulators involved induce changes in the pain pathways resulting in chronic pain for some patients. This is 1 reason that treating pain in the short term is important!

The initial pain-inducing event results in the activation of sensory nerve endings (by sodium) that take the signal up to the brain where brain areas related to nociception are activated: the somatosensory cortex, the amygdala, and others. Persistent or chronic pain results in remodeling of the brain in the corticolimbic system,* which affects the integration of our emotional responses—in this case, to pain.

There is a desperate need for alternatives to opiate pain management. Overdose of prescription opiates is the number 1 cause of death related to prescribed drugs. Both the ECS and endogenous opiate system (EOS) are known to be key systems in pain processing and immunomodulation, and crosstalk between these 2 systems is under investigation. The EOS is in high concentrations in the areas of the brain that produce analgesia, through inhibitory signals that travel down from the brain and inhibit pain signaling. Endorphins are sister compounds to the endocannabinoids because both are signaling all over the body, can be stimulated by exercise, sex, laughter, music, acupuncture, and meditation. They are also both associated with the experience called the runner's high. Both ECBs and endorphins participate in pain control, and are considered to be part of our body's feel-good hormones.[279] Activation of CB2R facilitates the release of beta-endorphin.[280, 281]

There are 4 main concepts of ECS/EOS crosstalk:[282, 283]

1. Both are key endogenous systems that exert control on several of the same physiologic effects: acting as sedatives, regulating pain sensation, involved in pain propagation, regulation of temperature, and regulation of intestinal motility.
2. Cannabinoids enhance the pain-relieving benefit of opiates and vice versa.
3. Administration of cannabinoid/opiate combinations show greater than additive effects in pain control.
4. The 2 systems are colocalized in the brain and on the immune cells that accumulate in damaged tissues or nerves.

Overdose of prescription opiates is the number one cause of death related to prescribed drugs. There is growing public perception that cannabis is

---

* The corticolimbic brain areas are involved in integrating emotion and cognition. The circuits in this brain network are associated with the emotional response to pain.

an effective pain therapy, while precise mechanisms, particularly synergy between cannabinoids and opioids, are not well understood.

It has been recorded in ancient texts of Chinese medicine that cannabis was also a component of an herbal formula along with opium used for anesthesia. The pathology of pain is likely disrupting ECS and EOS signaling, which explains why modulating both of these can help to resolve pain. By targeting both CB1R, for dampening the transmission of pain signals to the brain and altering perception of pain in the brain, and CB2R to dampen the inflammatory component of pain (THC activates both receptors), many people can achieve some analgesia or pain relief; some report complete resolution. As with any drug or therapy, there is a spectrum of results across individuals.

Plasticity in the brain is associated with chronic pain. The brain will adapt to the sensory input from the body and change signaling based on usage (like carving a rut in a road). The cortical area of the brain (somatosensory) that corresponds to the sensation coming from different parts of the body will adapt based on the amount of sensory input from that area of the body. Over time, if pain does not resolve due to healing of the tissue and nerves, there can be a transition to a chronic pain state, called central sensitization. In other words, the body forgets to stop feeling pain.

Neuroinflammation and activation of glial cells in the brain are both involved in this transition to chronic pain. What people with chronic pain experience includes:

- Allodynia: Experience pain with a stimulus that would not normally be painful (such as clothing touching the skin)
- Hyperalgesia: The pain sensation being exaggerated or more painful that it should be.

Opioids, used in the long term to address pain, have been shown to induce hyperalgesia.[284] Cannabis may help with both of these symptoms of chronic pain, along with allowing for the ability to shelve pain for a time, in order to get a better quality of life. CB2 receptor is another target for treating pain but this is less well understood than the CB1R targeting for pain.[285, 286]

Combining opioids with cannabis (at therapeutic dosing levels) may boost effects of both of these drugs, meaning that they work in synergy.[287] Cannabis was not shown to increase the level of opioids in the blood, which could lead to an overdose, and won't increase the likelihood of dying from an overdose when used together because the CB1R is not highly expressed in the brain stem.[288] Opioid receptors are in the brainstem, where they can shut down the heart and breathing. Simply removing opioids can provide significant pain improvement, after an initial amplification of pain as a withdrawal symptom.

Cannabis can be an herbal ally in this situation, or a harm-reduction approach, by helping to reduce the opioid dose, to prolong the time between doses (used in between opioid doses) and as an aid in tapering (reducing) opioid doses. Some people may be able to withdraw from opioid medications altogether, while others may be able to reduce the opioid dose and alleviate the hyperalgesia.[289] Long-term effects of opioid use on health include effects on cognitive function, immune and hormonal dysfunction, delayed gastric emptying, constipation, osteoporosis, and sleep disruption—all of which rob us of health.[290, 291] Medical science is demonstrating that cannabis is relatively safe and an effective pain reliever. In New York State, patients with legal access to cannabis were shown to reduce their use of prescription opioid medications.[292]

Neuropathic Pain

Mechanical damage to nerves causes a specific pain that involves all of the pain information processing pathways, from skin and muscles to spinal cord and the brain or the somatosensory system. It often manifests as shooting and burning pain and often becomes chronic. It tends to be progressive and is considered a chronic disease that affects up to 10% of the population. People with this diagnosis commonly have pain resulting from what would be a non-painful stimulus for most people, such as light touching, and associated with sleep disturbance, depression anxiety and impaired quality of life. This pain can occur after having a stroke, spinal cord injury, brain disease such as MS, cancer pain, herpes infections, HIV infection, diabetes, and damage to nerves from surgery or chemotherapy. Diabetes is a common reason for people to develop neuropathic pain where it may appear with a glove-and-stocking distribution as the forearms, hand, calves, and feet are prominently affected. It is challenging to treat this type of pain, particularly the hypersensitivity to stimuli, such as touch, heat, and cold. Alterations in ion channels (sodium, calcium, chloride) are involved and lead to increased excitability of these sensory signals.

The brain remodeling that co-occurs with chronic neuropathic pain include the amygdala and the anterior cingulate cortex, as these areas are intended to modulate the descending pain inhibition pathways. Signaling through serotonin and norepinephrine are implicated and this is why people with this type of pain may be placed on antidepressant medications (SSRIs or SNRIs) in addition to non-opioid pain medications like Lyrica or gabapentin, which modulate sodium channels and thereby neuronal excitability.[293]

Benzodiazepines are also prescribed to treat the anxiety/emotional aspect of pain. It was reported in early 2023 that increased frequency of benzodiazepine use was associated with pain intensity,[294] underscoring that this drug needs to be closely watched in people with pain as there can be an increase in pain catastrophizing.

CB1R can be downregulated with extended use of opioid medications; using cannabis as a means to upregulate the ECS again is a strategy for helping with neuropathic pain. Starting with low doses of THC and building to personal tolerance can particularly help with the hypersensitivity to sensations that should not be painful (allodynia). The upregulation of CB2R on microglia is another potential therapeutic mechanism by which cannabis may help with pain, as this increase in the CB2R is another gating element that promotes pain. Inflammatory pain signals can be dampened by targeting the activation of this receptor.

Complex Regional Pain Syndrome (CRPS)

Also known reflex sympathetic dystrophy (RSD), CRPS is a condition in which chronic, intense pain (often in one arm, leg, hand, or foot) worsens over time and spreads in the affected area. These conditions are typically accompanied by color or temperature changes of the skin where the pain is felt. The pain is usually initiated by tissue damage such as from surgery, fracture, or blunt trauma; it more commonly affects women. This is a debilitating condition, often unrelieved by any existing therapies. There is a strong inflammatory component to this pain disorder, which can be helped by steroid drugs (prednisone), but this is not sustainable in the long term. This is another situation where there is sensitization to pain due to the changes in the pain pathways in the brain. Many of these patients may be put on anti-convulsant drugs, gabapentin, amitriptyline (known as a tricyclic antidepressant), and some other drug cocktails. Ketamine is another therapeutic approach, and more recently the plant *Psilocybe* (species usually *cubensis*) is being tried.

Movement Disorders

The first description of cannabis to treat muscle spasms was in the writings of Arab Muslim philosopher Abū Yūsuf al-Kindī in the 9th century BCE. Almost 1,000 years later, cannabis extracts were still being reported to have an effect on muscle contraction in the treatment of tetanus in India, reported to improve survival. Because of the location of the ECS in the centers of the brain that control movement, drugs that inhibit anandamide hydrolysis result in decreased locomotor and exploratory activity. When the body forgets to stop moving as with tremor, dyskinesia, epilepsy, spasms, RLS, and tics, targeting the ECS may be a means of treating these disorders. In addition, the neuroprotective effects of plant cannabinoids may help to protect the brain from damage caused by the overactivity in brain centers that are hyperreactive in these situations.

Parkinson's Disease

The use of tincture of Indian hemp (squire's extract) to treat the tremor of PD was first described by British neurologist Sir William Gowers in his landmark textbook published in the late 19th century.[295] The effects of cannabis in PD are related to a group of structures at the center of the brain called the basal ganglia that contains an abundance of CB receptors. Therefore, it is not surprising that cannabinoids have significant effects on the control of voluntary movement, as this is the brain region that sends signals to your muscles, telling them to move (motor function). PD is the second most common neurological disease (after AD), with estimates of 9 million cases by 1930, worldwide. PD can be associated with both motor and non-motor symptoms as well as behavioral, emotional, depression, anxiety, and insomnia components.

Cannabinoids and AEA are interacting with three major neurotransmitters in the basal ganglia: dopamine, GABA, and glutamate. Anandamide levels in blood have been measured to be twice as high of that in healthy people. DA is the major neurotransmitter produced by neurons located in the area known as the substantia nigra (SN) important for both movement and reward. Neurons in these regions with DA receptors are part of a network of neuronal feedback loops critical for the normal execution of the programming for movement. PD results in the gradual loss of DA neurons of the SN. The loss of DA is responsible for the gradual manifestation and progression of physical symptoms including slow imprecise movements (bradykinesia), tremors at rest, rigidity, facial paucity (hypomimia), shuffling gait, difficulty walking, freezing, and postural instability.[296] Slowness of movement and rigidity could be thought of as forgetting to move, while tremor might be the opposite. Different symptom sets appear across patients.

It is known that the CB1Rs are colocalized with 2 dopamine receptors, D1 and D2. Activation of the CB1R with an agonist inhibits both the D1R and D2R—this may explain why there is a decrease in locomotor activity and sedation noted in animals given THC. On the other hand, activation of the CB1R inhibits DA reuptake, and can potentiate the effects of DA. CB1R has been shown to be downregulated in the brains of patients with PD, but levodopa* may help to upregulate the receptor.[297] Drugs that specifically inhibit DA reuptake (dopamine transporter blockers like cocaine) increase motor activity but can also produce anxiety and addictive behaviors. The paradoxical effects may seem difficult to understand, but the consensus

---

* Levodopa is a precursor to dopamine used to treat symptoms of dopamine insufficiency.

is that stimulation of CB1R by cannabinoid agonists is important for the long-term modulation of DA neurotransmission.

Cannabis was rarely recommended for treatment of PD in the 20th century primarily because of societal and legal restrictions. However, there are many anecdotal reports on the usefulness of cannabis preparations for treatment of symptoms of PD and for alleviation of the involuntary movements (dyskinesias) that often plague patients who take levodopa (an oral form of dopamine) for treatment of PD. The frequency of self-medication with cannabis in the US is not known, but a survey of PD patients in the Czech Republic revealed a significant proportion of respondents to a questionnaire were using cannabis to help treat symptoms of PD.[298] Most of the patients reported using about 1/2 teaspoon of cannabis flower orally, usually in food. Only 1 patient smoked the cannabis.

Almost half reported mild/substantial help with PD symptoms: 30% with improvement of resting tremor, 45% alleviation of bradykinesia, 38% alleviation of muscle rigidity, and (14%) improvement of L-dopa-induced dyskinesias. In a small component of this study, a cannabinoid assay was performed on the urine samples donated from patients. This revealed that it was high levels of THC (>50 ng/mL) associated with improvement in bradykinesia or rigidity, whereas those with low levels of THC metabolite had no improvement in either slowness or rigidity. These levels in the blood are more often associated with inhalation of cannabis, rather than taking orally. Self-medication with cannabis appeared to be beneficial in a significant number of these patients. While findings from questionnaires have many limitations and are not conclusive, they can provide some evidence for cannabis and quality of life in PD. Some patients with PD also have pain, for which cannabis can be helpful.[299]

As insomnia is a prominent feature in PD, cannabis has the potential to help PD patients conserve their cognitive health by promoting sleep.[300] The original description of PD, published in 1817 by the neurologist Dr. James Parkinson, stated that: "Tremulous motions of the limbs occur during sleep, and augment until they awaken the patient, and frequently with much agitation and alarm."[301] This is now known as REM sleep behavior disorder (RBD). Some patients with PD suffer from RBD, associated with nightmares, wild movement of limbs, shouting (which indicates a dysfunction in circadian function), and sleep architecture that Dr. Parkinson described. In fact, 74% of people with RBD were diagnosed a neurodegenerative disease within 12 years of having RBD diagnosed.[302]

There are also likely neuroprotective effects of cannabinoids to help slow loss of dopaminergic neurons. CBD and THC are both candidates for the neuroprotective effects, but THC is more likely to have effects on sleep quality. The PD brain needs to have the nightly sweeping to prevent accumulation of a protein called alpha-synuclein. This protein is the hallmark of Lewy bodies, which is indicative of Lewy body dementia. These proteins in the brain aggregate and deposit in (also in AD and in Huntington disease) in the DA neurons (assisted by damage from ROS, see Chapter Eat) where these deposits are toxic to cells. The only available treatments for PD and other proteinopathies are to manage symptoms.

Cannabinoids are antioxidant and may be protective in this setting, along with other phytochemicals.[303] Binding the CB2R, accomplished by THC and many dietary cannabinoids, is critical for modulating the effects of inflammation that are associated with dopaminergic neuron damage and death.[304] Sources for plant compounds that bind CB2 are reviewed in Chapter 4: Protect, along with dietary antioxidants and anti-inflammatories. Lion's mane mushroom contains a compound that may be protective in the case of cognitive effects in PD.[305]

Epilepsy

Epilepsy is the most common neurological disorder that affects around 50 million people worldwide. Seizures are the principal symptom of epilepsy, a chronic and sometimes progressive disorder due to excessive neuronal activity—often with an unknown cause. Approximately 30% of individuals with epilepsy do not obtain adequate seizure control from existing drugs, some of which can themselves cause debilitating and life-threatening side effects. Up to 50% of people with epilepsy ultimately develop seizures that are resistant to medicines. These factors drive both patient and commercial searches for more effective and better-tolerated therapies, which may include *Cannabis*. In general, activation of the CB1R reduces the severity of seizure in mouse models; increasing ECB levels is another experimental strategy. Low-serum AEA has been measured in patient with temporal lobe epilepsy.[306] Similar to THC, AEA may have biphasic effects whereby high concentrations may cause seizures. This may be due to the activation of TRPV1 receptor at higher concentrations.

The use of *Cannabis* for seizure control was described by Arabic pioneer in psychosomatic medications, Ali ibn al-Mayusi (circa 1100 BCE), Ibn al-Badri in the 15th century, and by medical practitioners in the 1800s.[,307-309] *Cannabis* use has been reported to have both proconvulsant and anticonvulsant effects. CBD is the only other phytocannabinoid investigated for anticonvulsant effects in human subjects.[310] There is now an FDA-approved drug, Epidiolex, for treating this patient population.

Intractable epilepsy (IE) of childhood, such as Dravet Syndrome (a mutation in a calcium channel), occurs in about 3% of the population and is generally associated with frequent, treatment-resistant seizure, poor quality of life, and developmental delay. There are various known clinical diagnoses of IE of childhood, and as many of unknown etiology. Antiepileptic drugs (AEDs) attempt to modulate or block a number of receptors, but children's seizures are resistant to all of the drugs in the conventional neurology toolkit. The approach of using cannabinoids took this community by storm around 2009.[311] I started working with these families in 2010.

A group of 30 families elected to start their children with diagnoses of IE on a CBD-dominant whole plant extract that was provided at no charge by a cannabis company in Washington State. A cannabis chemotype known as ACDC (the father of a patient of mine brought these clones back to Washington after acquiring them from the breeder in Northern California) was grown in an indoor-grow facility and was quality-control tested after extraction with ethanol and evaporation that produced a solid extract (SE) of the cannabis. Analytical results showed that across samples and harvests/batches, the product was consistent with 82.5% CBD and 4% THC content for a total of 907 mg of CBD and 44 mg of THC per 1.1 gram vial that was distributed to the parent.

Working with some of the parents, we collaboratively developed a work-sheet to help parents define dosing This was based on a treatment protocol first used in my private practice in early 2012. The protocol provided for an upward titration dose of CBD starting with of 0.5 mg/kg of the child's weight. The parent would enter the child's weight in kilograms, the % CBD/THC of the batch of SE they were using, and then how many milliliters of food-grade oil (such as olive, hemp, macadamia, coconut) to add to the SE for a specific mg dose was calculated. They usually gave it to their child 3 times a day. They were instructed to slowly increase the dose by 0.5 mL every 3–7 days, based on the child's tolerance (watching for sedation, gas-trointestinal problems, increase in seizure). The parents continued to up-wardly titrate the dose looking for the lowest, most effective target dose possible. All of the families reported that their child was more alert, more verbal and sleeping better, while 6 families observed better mood and im-proved gross or fine motor skills.

There was an average of 50% reduction in how often seizure occurred and they reported that the children were recovering faster from the post-ictal phase. Seizure reduction and decreased severity of seizure may also corre-late with more rapid recovery in the postictal phase. It has been reported that seizure damages dendrites and this plays a role in the postictal phase, after a seizure resolves. Instead of removing the structure, in this case mi-croglia seem to be providing a supportive role by protecting the dendrites by wrapping around them to stabilize them rather than engulfing them act-ing as neuroprotectants (see Protect).

The most notable anecdotes from parents were comments that indicated that they felt as if they were meeting their child for the first time. The de-scriptions "awakening" and "coming to life" were used as well as reports of the children talking more. One family reported their son rode his bike after not having ridden for 2 years. One child ate 2 meals when she had only previously been fed by G-tube. Another child pronounced her name for the first time in 8 years. One child who had previously had 20 tonic-clonic seizures a day had experienced seizure only on 7 days of the previous 3 months. I reported this at the International Cannabinoid Research Society meeting in Italy 2018 and there was barely a dry eye in the room.[312] The available literature (case studies, surveys, and preclinical data) on the use of *Cannabis* or individual cannabinoids for the treatment of epilepsy and seizures in humans suggests that *Cannabis* exerts an anticonvulsant effect, and rarely acts as a proconvulsant.

Brain Tumors

Cancer in general is a state of the body's immune system forgetting to eliminate mutated cells. This is not all the fault of the immune system, as these rogue cells have found ways to hide from the immune cells that would destroy them. The earlier a cluster of cancer cells is caught by laboratory or imaging studies, the better the chance of treating and resolving the cancer. In the 1940s, the first results of chemotherapy treatment were published, showing reduction in the size of tumors in people with lymphoma. These drugs come at a cost however since they are not capable of differentiating healthy cells that are rapidly dividing from tumor cells that are rapidly dividing. This results in the side effects of chemotherapy including nausea/vomiting, appetite loss, diarrhea, hair loss, fatigue, fever, nerve damage, and mouth sores. Cannabis has been used to help stimulate appetite and helping food taste better, deter weight loss by taking in more calories, treat pain associated with tumors or nerve pain from chemotherapy, and help with anxiety and sleep. One agent, cannabis, could potentially replace a number of drugs, each one targeting a different symptom![313] I authored a paper on this topic that was published by the National Cancer Institute in their *Cannabis* monograph in 2021.[ ]

There are a number of studies suggesting that cancer growth could be inhibited by cannabinoids.[314, 315] They way that they do this is induction of apoptosis in tumor cells.* Cannabinoids may also slow cell growth (antiproliferative) and slow the spread of cells to other areas of the body (antimetastatic) by stopping the blood supply to tumors and slowing the migration of the tumor cells, and even cell death. Some of these actions of

---

* Apoptosis is the process of a cell self-destructing due to internal sensors in the cell signaling that is a normal part of homeostasis of the organism. It is known as programmed cell death.

cannabinoids were first shown in brain tumor cells, which makes sense because neuronal cells will be expressing CBRs (not all tumor cells have CBRs).

Other cell lines that have been studied to respond to cannabinoids are leukemia/lymphoma, neuroblastoma, uterine, breast, gastric, colorectal, pancreatic, and prostate carcinomas. The cell-killing potential was first demonstrated in glioma cells where the mechanism described to be responsible for cell death is a process called autophagy, a process upstream of mitochondria by which the cell may destroy itself or damaged/abnormal parts of itself. However, these results may not translate directly to human cancers, particularly when in the situation where any cancer is advanced. I am regularly contacted by people hoping for some type of Hail Mary cure for a loved one's cancer, but most cancers are the most treatable when caught early, and when treated using up-to-date scientific approaches. Since the time of early studies on cells, THC has been tried as a therapy for the devastating brain tumor called glioblastoma (GBM), a system invasion of the brain by tumor cells.[316]

In a pilot study, THC was injected directly into the tumor site of patients with GBM where it was reported to be well-tolerated, but unfortunately none of the patients survived.[317] The average time of survival after GBM diagnosis is about 1 year. This study did suggest that THC could be helpful, particularly if it was administered along with the chemotherapy drug temozolomide. The drug Sativex was given to patients, either 6 or 7.5 sprays/day (2.5 mg CBD and 2.7 mg THC per spray).[318] The overall survival of patients who received both chemotherapy and Sativex was better than those with chemotherapy alone, but this was in a small number of patients.

This was the first study of its type, suggesting that giving cannabis with chemo is a viable approach; however, it is not always well-tolerated by cancer patients. In my clinical experience, and in this study, these patients are usually not tolerant to the THC side effects and it can worsen balance, dizziness, and increase heart rate, as well as cause nausea and constipation for some. Many people with cancer try cannabis either for palliative symptoms or to try to treat tumors. The important thing is whether or not the tumor has the CBRs, because if the target is not there, then there will be no potential for inhibiting the tumor cells. While research indicates some compounds in cannabis can inhibit the growth of cancerous cells, that doesn't mean it's a cure. Cancer patients who rely on cannabis to treat their condition can face potential health risks and the reports on killing of cancer cells should not be taken out of context. The very high doses that would likely be required to lead to cell death can be debilitating for some people. See Box 5.4 for actions to take if experiencing negative acute cannabis effects

Naturopathic/Integrative/Functional Approaches
Toning the ECS

If you are interested in toning DMN activity, then mindfulness-based meditation is your friend! Mindfulness is considered to be an individual's ability or tendency to consciously engage in a state of non-judgmental awareness to the present moment.[319] Training in mindfulness may help to tone the DMN, as those who are regular meditators had different signals between the DMN regions compared to those who do not meditate.[320] This means training in mindfulness could be helpful in helping the brain to refocus and not wander into stressful scenarios. Research into this area is a hot topic due to its potential effects on anxiety, depression, ADHD, OCD, stress reduction, and pain. The hypothesis is that mindfulness may work in part by increasing the DMN and the SN connectivity meaning that meditators become more aware of mind wandering or self-thoughts.

Terpene

Pinene is the most abundant of the monoterpenes and is reported to inhibit the breakdown of acetylcholine.[321] This leads to more acetylcholine left unmetabolized and available to bind its receptor. This is the same strategy of drug therapy for treating cognitive dysfunction in dementia and AD. Pinene is abundant in essential oils of pine and rosemary. If you have ever walked into a pine forest, you have experienced the mind-clearing effects of pinene. This terpene may also act as an anti-inflammatory and increase glutathione. Pinene seems to have largely been bred out of cannabis species. Blue Dream is a classic chemotype where pinene content at least equaled myrcene, overriding the sedating property of myrcene. When dry vaped, the effects include mental and physical stimulation, creativity, inspiration, and invigoration. Pinene is likely behind the effects of 'sativa' type of cannabis experience. Terpinoline may have similar effects as that of pinene.

Measuring Allostatic Load

You can measure AL using neurofilament light (as a measure of blood-brain-barrier function), glutathione, DHEAs, homocysteine, lipid panels for HDL-C, triglycerides, and LDLs (types are important).

Neurofeedback is a noninvasive approach using technology for real-time EEG that monitors your brain wave activity, presents it as feedback to you, then allows you to self-regulate brain activity and train your brain. This type of reinforcement learning has been shown to have beneficial effects on cognitive processes, anxiety, pain, PTSD, and ADHD inferred from behavior.

Exercise

Any exercise is good for the brain—even daily walking is recommended for older people to reduce the risk of dementia by 30%. To combat effects of resistance to insulin post-menopausally, high intensity interval training (HIIT) or short intensity training (SIT) activate short twitch muscles. For bone health, either impact (such as walking or running) or weight/strength training can help to prevent fractures. Pilates is a great way to burn fat and increase strength.

Herbal Allies

Humulus lupulus (hops) is a cousin plant to cannabis and also contains a group of compounds unique to this plant called prenylated chalcones and also flavonoids. Hops contains a compound, xanthohumol, that is suggested to have anticancer effects.[322] You don't have to drink hops in beer; I make my own kombucha with hops or you can make it into a tea. In addition to the calming and sedative effects, by using hops you may be boosting anti-cancer mechanisms (preventing damage to DNA) in your body.[323] Xanthohumol can be taken as a supplement also. Usually in the process of making beer, these compounds are lost by being converted to flavanones. Different

BOX 5.4 WHAT TO DO IF YOU HAVE NEGATIVE SIDE EFFECTS FROM CANNABIS

1) FAST HEARTBEAT: An increase in heart rate may feel like anxiety or a panic attack. If you experience this, remain seated and employ one of the following breathing techniques:

PURSED LIP BREATHING: Breathe out for double the amount of breathing in. Sitting up as straight as you can, with relaxed shoulders, take a normal breath for about 4 counts. Then pucker your lips up (think of your mouth when you're about to whistle—that's what your lips should look like!) and exhale for 8 counts. Repeat for 6–8 breaths.

DIAPHRAGMATIC BREATHING: Breathe through your nose and focus on how your belly fills up with air. You can do this one either sitting up very straight or lying down. With your shoulders back, keep one hand on your chest and the other on your belly. As you breathe in deeply for about 4–6 seconds, your belly should stick out a bit. Feel the air expanding your stomach and then breathe out slowly, feeling your stomach contract, for a count of 8–12 seconds using the pursed lips as in the first exercise.

2) DIZZINESS: This may occur upon rising from a seated or lying down position as a result of blood-pressure reducing effects of THC, when inhaled. Try to prevent this by being well hydrated, rising slowly from being seated, and also by employing the breathing exercises previously described.

3) FEELING SLEEPY: It's okay if you feel sleepy and want to lie down to nap. If you don't want to do this, then consider engaging in light exercise, such as going on a walk or performing stretching exercises.

4) DRY MOUTH: Drinking fluids can help, or chewing gum or sucking a hard candy.

5) DISSOCIATIVE SYMPTOMS: This is a feeling where you think you are an outside observer with respect to your thoughts, body, and sensations. Some people describe this as feeling heady. Engaging in an activity where you are not focusing on your thoughts can be helpful, such as arts/crafts, listening to music, singing ,and dancing to music, watching an entertaining show, or having a friend to talk to.

6) ANXIETY: Beyond the potential elevation in heart rate, THC can activate the part of your brain that stores memories causing recall of thoughts around events that may be distressing. If this happens:

A) Always go back to the breathing exercises described above.

B) Remind yourself that you are not in any danger and tell yourself: "I'm safe. This will pass. I'll feel better soon."

C) Use grounding techniques, which are intended to bring you back into the present moment, by engaging your physical senses. Grounding is not about making the feeling go away as much as staying present in your body while noticing your thoughts. Here are some examples of grounding activities:

BATHE: Take a shower or bath. Switching the shower from warm to cold can enhance this. This is a form of self-soothing.

EAT: Savor some food that sounds good to you. Take small bites of a favorite food or sip some hot tea and indulge in the sensory experience.

EXERCISE: Yoga is a good method for this. Using rhythm can also be helpful, so turning on music and moving to the beat or even just tapping your feet can give you a focus.

SMELL: Indulge in a scent that you love. This could be essential oils, candles, or a cup of tea. Inhale the fragrance and focus on the quality of the scent.

SOUND: Listen to the ambient sounds around you, or put on a podcast, music or audiobook.

COMPANIONSHIP: Spend time with a friend, family member, or pet.

NATURE: Indulge the senses by going outside, to a park, or the beach. Focus on the things around you in all of their detail.

DISTRACTION: Do an activity that requires engaging your body: gardening, knitting, washing dishes, folding laundry, cooking, or cleaning the kitchen.

HERE IS THE 54321 TECHNIQUE IF YOU FEEL OVERWHELMED OR ANXIOUS:

5: ACKNOWLEDGE **5** things you see around you. It could be a pen, a spot on the ceiling, or anything else in your surroundings.

4: ACKNOWLEDGE **4** things you can touch around you. It could be your hair, a pillow, or the ground under your feet.

3: ACKNOWLEDGE **3** things you hear. This could be any external sound. If you can hear your belly rumbling, that counts! Focus on things you can hear outside of your body.

2: ACKNOWLEDGE **2** things you can smell. Maybe you are in your office and smell pencil, or maybe you are in your bedroom and smell a pillow. Take a brief walk to find a scent or smell soap in your bathroom.

1: ACKNOWLEDGE **1** thing you can taste. What does the inside of your mouth taste like—gum, coffee, or the sandwich from lunch?

types of hops will contain differing amounts of xanthohumol. Hops have been used traditionally across cultures for problems such as liver disease, foot odor, leprosy, sleep disturbance, and constipation in addition to the imbibement joy when in a fermented form (beer). If you are going to drink beer, drink a strong hoppy imperial pale ale to get the most hops; better yet, make kombucha with hops!

Hericium erinaceus: Lion's mane is an edible mushroom found growing wild in North America from August to November, which grows on dead trees. It contains some diverse phytochemicals, the polysaccharides that are immune-boosting, but also hericenones and erinacines. Hericenones and erinacines, specifically erinacine A, have been found to promote the synthesis of NGF and BDNF. Erinacine A is only found in the mycelium, but not the fruiting body, so choose your product wisely! Eating them is good for you, too.

Trametes versicolor: Turkey tail mushroom grows all over the world and is a woody type of mushroom. A polysaccharide from turkey tail has been used as an adjuvant in the treatment of breast cancers and immune deficiencies. Polysaccharo-peptide has been shown to upregulate CB2R expression, which may help with pain control by increasing the levels of beta-endorphin and activating the mu-opioid receptors. Upregulation of CB2R can also impact brain health by subsequent binding of the receptor with dietary cannabinoid, thereby decreasing inflammation in the brain. Either an alcohol extract or the mycelium is suggested for intake.[324-326]

Cinnamomum verum: Cinnamon studies suggest that this dried bark of the cinnamon tree has anti-inflammatory, antioxidant, and anticancer properties, and can also boost the immune system. A number of compounds have been identified that could positively alter cognitive function such as eugenol, cinnamaldehyde, and cinnamic acid. While primarily used as a spice, it is one of the most potent antioxidants in the spice world! Use it liberally. It may also help to stabilize blood sugar and lower HbA1c (a marker for metabolic disease).

Magnolia grandiflora L.: (Magnolia bark) contains compounds that act as both CB2R modulator and COX-2 substrate-specific inhibitor (both anti-inflammatory pathways) and has shown beneficial effects in animal models of neurodegeneration. Magnolia bark is known for helping with relaxation and pain, and boosting mood. Tetrahydromagnolol is a major metabolite of one of the main bioactive phytochemicals in magnolia bark. It has been used in traditional Chinese and Japanese medicine to treat pain. Remember that treating inflammation can help with cognitive health.

Angelica sinensis: Dong qui is one of the most widely used medicines in Chinese medicine formularies.* It has traditionally been used for gynecological problems, in formulas with other botanicals, as with most Chinese medicine (rather than a single agent). It is thought to be a good blood tonic, and has been studied for use in acute stroke because it is known to stimulate circulation and inhibit platelet aggregation. Its most important use has been for treating menstrual disorders such as painful menstruation, endometriosis, and uterine fibroids. It has been shown to relax smooth muscles (spasmolytic), so may have benefits both on the uterus and the blood vessels for high blood pressure (this must be from an alcohol-based extract). The compound ligustilide is thought to be responsible for these effects. It also has potential estrogenic effects and may be supportive of menopause in this way. A clinic study did not show it to have pro-estrogenic effects on the lining of the uterus.

Food/Nutrition/Diet**

The Mediterranean diet and the DASH (dietary approaches to stop hypertension) intervention for neurodegenerative delay (MIND) diet may be helpful in preventing or delaying Alzheimer's disease or other age-related

---

* The America Herbal Pharmacopoeia (AHP) is a nonprofit organization that has published monographs on many botanical medicines since 1996. The early pharmacopoeias that included plants ended in about 1936 in favor of synthetic drugs, changing the nature of medicine. You can find detailed information about many herbal medicines through this organization: https://herbal-ahp.org/.

** The National Institutes of Health publishes updated information on this topic: https://www.nia.nih.gov/health/what-do-we-know-about-diet-and-prevention-alzheimers-disease.

cognitive decline. Eating a fresh, whole foods diet helps to reduce oxidative stress, reduce blood pressure, prevent diabetes, obesity, and heart disease. Getting plenty of fiber also supports the gut microbiome. The MIND diet limits servings of red meat, sweets, cheese, butter/margarine, and fast/fried food:

- Leafy green vegetables, at least 6 servings/week
- Other vegetables, at least 1 serving/day
- Berries, at least 2 servings/week
- Whole grains, at least 3 servings/day
- Fish, 1 serving/week
- Poultry, 2 servings/week
- Beans, 3 servings/week
- Nuts, 5 servings/week
- Olive oil

Omega-3s: A major substrate for inflammatory compounds made in the body is AA, the same fatty acid that ECBs are derived from. A-beta in a normal concentration may act as an anti-inflammatory, but when there is an excess of a-beta and fatty acids are biased toward having an abundance of AA, this is a toxic situation for nerve cells.[ ] Cannabinoids may be protective in this setting, but shifting our fatty acid balance is important for nerve health. A supplement of fish oil at 2,000 grams twice per day is what I suggest for anti-inflammatory benefit not only for the brain but for joint health and bone health.

Supplements

Lithium orotate: Lithium is an essential micromineral that is primarily accessed through our water supply. Many geographical areas are deficient in lithium, which leads to deficiency in humans. Decreased levels of lithium in drinking water are associated with increased incidence of a host of harmful mood-related conditions.[327] Hair lithium levels are low in certain pathological conditions (eg, heart disease) in learning-disabled subjects and in incarcerated violent criminals.

Orotate is a carrier molecule that helps to transport lithium into cells.[328] This form of lithium is not the same as what is given by prescription to treat bipolar disorder (lithium salts), but is an over-the-counter nutritional supplement. The supplement form works well to help manage mood disturbances, in my clinical experience, helping with anxiety and hypomanic behavior. It acts by inhibiting GSK3b, and aberrant activity of this protein is linked to the disruption of circadian function, impaired neurogenesis, decreased expression of neurotrophic factors, and hyperactivity in humans. Treating with lithium may help to rescue BDNF, normalize inositol levels in the brain, and attenuate neuroinflammation.[329]

Magnesium: There is a protective role for magnesium in neurological diseases including headache, TBI, PD, and AD. The best form for getting magnesium into the brain is magnesium threonate (MagT). High doses of this form can be given without causing the gastrointestinal effects of other forms of magnesium (diarrhea usually happens for most people at about 200 mg dose). MagT may also help improve memory functions by upregulation of NMDA receptor.[330]

Zinc: Deficiency in this mineral is associated with endoplasmic reticulum function and associated with protein misfolding. Oysters have the highest level of zinc compared to other seafoods, meats, and food in general. Don't take too much though, as it can deplete copper at too high of a concentration; 11 mg/day is the recommended daily allowance.

mTOR Inhibitors: Mechanistic target of rapamycin (mTOR) regulates cell growth, proliferation, synthesis of lipids, and the translation of proteins. Cancer, obesity, diabetes, and some skin conditions have altered mTOR regulation. It is also involved in the pathogenesis of AD. Inhibiting the signaling of mTOR is an approach for aging and disease; there are natural products that have been studied to perform this service:

- Curcumin is the yellow pigment found in turmeric, is anti-inflammatory, and has been shown to arrest cell growth.
- Resveratrol is a naturally occurring pigment found in grapes, cranberries, and peanuts.

- Caffeine is an alkaloid found in coffee, tea, and cocoa beans. Epigal-locatechin-3-gallate is the most abundant phytochemical in green tea.[331]

BDNF Boosters

- Moderate-intensity exercise several times per week
- Controlling stress levels by saying no and having a good tool kit for stress resilience
- Combating inflammation with diet, lifestyle, and phytochemicals that are anti-inflammatory
- Calorie restriction, especially carbohydrates
- Supplementation with CBD

Glutathione: This is our body's most potent antioxidant and is known to be depleted in the brain in both in the early stages of PD and in AD.[332] It may even be considered to be a biomarker of AD and MCI or of the oxidative stress related to aging in general! It is a small molecule made of cysteine, glycine, and glutamic acid. Our body makes it in the liver and in the brain in high amounts, and it can be recycled. To make glutathione, you have to have plenty of cysteine and supplementation with N-acetyl-cysteine (NAC) is one way to do this (orally or by IV). There are also glutathione supplements, but the stomach acid may break the molecule down into its 3 components. Giving glutathione intranasally is another strategy and it has been shown to get directly into the brain.[333] Deficiency of this essential antioxidant has been shown to perpetuate oxidative stress, resulting in cell death and dysfunction of mitochondria.

Nicotinamide adenine dinucleotide (NAD): NAD is an essential compo-nent of cellular functioning because it carries electrons in the mitochondrial generation of energy. While our body makes NAD, lack of niacin in the diet can lead to depletion of this important compound. It is used by SIRT1 (dis-cussed earlier). NAD is not very stable taken orally, but using a supplement of niacinamide will suffice and will allow to bypass the flushing that occurs with niacin. A growing body of evidence supports that boosting cellular levels of NAD may confer neuroprotective effects in both healthy aging and neurodegeneration. Enhancing the replenishment of this molecule could potentially help to ameliorate processes implicated in the pathogenesis of PD, including mitochondrial respiratory dysfunction. Taken orally at 500 mg twice per day, NAD was shown to get into the brain.[334]

CDP Choline: Citicoline is the form of the nutrient choline that I recommend for supplementation; it has high bioavailability. CDP choline is a nootropic compound (cognitive enhancer) that crosses the BBB and increases cerebral metabolism and helps to support neurotransmitter synthesis that may help with attention, focus and memory. The recommended dose is 500 mg/day.

Chakra/Yoga

The fifth chakra or vishuddhas is associated anatomically with the cervical plexus of nerves and the thyroid gland. The color associated with this chakra is turquoise. It is about inspiration, expression, creative energy and governs our self-expression and communication. Yoga postures associated with this chakra include sarvangasana (shoulder stand), halasana (plough pose), and setu bandha sarvangasana (bridge pose). Chanting the eternal sound "om" activates this chakra. Make it a long, slow, resonating sound, ending with your lips together in the "mmmm" sound until you feel your chest vibrating. The jlandara bhanda or chin lock helps to bring energy to this chakra.

How Does THC or CBD Affect Your Cognitive Function?

Chart Your Results

Trials	Date/ Time	Oral/ Inhaled	Dose/ Product	Ability to Work	Ability to Read	Forgetfulness	Creativity
1							
2							
3							
4							

How Does THC or CBD Affect Your Pain?

Chart Your Results: score pain and quality of life **0-10** with 10 being the worst pain and 10 as the best quality of life

Trials	Date/ Time	Oral/ Inhaled	Dose/ Product	Pain rating before	Pain rating after	Sedation	Quality of life Before/After
1							
2							
3							
4							

References

1. Di Marzo, V., et al., *Endocannabinoids: endogenous cannabinoid receptor ligands with neuromodulatory action.* Trends Neurosci, 1998. **21**(12): p. 521-8.
2. Gaoni, Y.a.M., R, *Isolation, Structure, and Partial Synthesis of an Active Constituent of Hashish.* Journal of the American Chemical Society, 1954. **86**(8): p. 1646-1647.
3. Devane, W.A., et al., *Isolation and structure of a brain constituent that binds to the cannabinoid receptor.* Science, 1992. **258**(5090): p. 1946-9.
4. Mechoulam, R., et al., *Identification of an endogenous 2-monoglyceride, present in canine gut, that binds to cannabinoid receptors.* Biochem Pharmacol, 1995. **50**(1): p. 83-90.
5. Bramley, E.V., *The trauma doctor: Gabor. Mate on happiness, hope and how to heal our deepest wounds.*, in *The Guardian.* 2023, Guardian Media Group.
6. Lohr, J.B., et al., *Allostatic load and the cannabinoid system: implications for the treatment of physiological abnormalities in post-traumatic stress disorder (PTSD).* CNS Spectr, 2020. **25**(6): p. 743-749.
7. *Get your ACE Score.*
8. Aronow, W.S. and J. Cassidy, *Effect of marihuana and placebo-marihuana smoking on angina pectoris.* N Engl J Med, 1974. **291**(2): p. 65-7.
9. Renaud, A.M. and Y. Cormier, *Acute effects of marihuana smoking on maximal exercise performance.* Med Sci Sports Exerc, 1986. **18**(6): p. 685-9.
10. L., et al., *The effect of cannabinoids on the stretch reflex in multiple sclerosis spasticity.* Int Clin Psychopharmacol, 2016. **31**(4): p. 232-9.
11. Heyman, E., et al., *Intense exercise increases circulating endocannabinoid and BDNF levels in humans--possible implications for reward and depression.* Psychoneuroendocrinology, 2012. **37**(6): p. 844-51.
12. Thompson, Z., et al., *Circulating levels of endocannabinoids respond acutely to voluntary exercise, are altered in mice selectively bred for high voluntary wheel running, and differ between the sexes.* Physiol Behav, 2017. **170**: p. 141-150.
13. Raichlen, D.A., et al., *Exercise-induced endocannabinoid signaling is modulated by intensity.* Eur J Appl Physiol, 2013. **113**(4): p. 869-75.

14. Raichlen, D.A., et al., *Wired to run: exercise-induced endocannabinoid signaling in humans and cursorial mammals with implications for the 'runner's high'.* J Exp Biol, 2012. **215**(Pt 8): p. 1331-6.

15. Fride, E., *Cannabinoids and Feeding: The Role of the Endogenous Cannabinoid System as a Trigger for Newborn Suckling.* Journal of Cannabis Therapeutics, 2002. **2**(3-4): p. 51-62.

16. Price, C.J., E.A. Thompson, and S.C. Cheng, *Scale of Body Connection: A multi-sample construct validation study.* PLoS One, 2017. **12**(10): p. e0184757.

17. Cardinal, P., et al., *Hypothalamic CB1 cannabinoid receptors regulate energy balance in mice.* Endocrinology, 2012. **153**(9): p. 4136-43.

18. Koch, M., et al., *Hypothalamic POMC neurons promote cannabinoid-induced feeding.* Nature, 2015. **519**(7541): p. 45-50.

19. Kalant, O.J., *Report of the Indian Hemp Drugs Commission, 1893-94: a critical review.* Int J Addict, 1972. **7**(1): p. 77-96.

20. Espel-Huynh, H.M., A.F. Muratore, and M.R. Lowe, *A narrative review of the construct of hedonic hunger and its measurement by the Power of Food Scale.* Obes Sci Pract, 2018. **4**(3): p. 238-249.

21. Lowe, M.R., et al., *The Power of Food Scale. A new measure of the psychological influence of the food environment.* Appetite, 2009. **53**(1): p. 114-8.

22. Yoshida, R., et al., *Endocannabinoids selectively enhance sweet taste.* Proc Natl Acad Sci U S A, 2010. **107**(2): p. 935-9.

23. Keyshams, N., et al., *Cannabinoid-glutamate interactions in the regulation of food intake in neonatal layer- type chicks: role of glutamate NMDA and AMPA receptors.* Vet Res Commun, 2016. **40**(2): p. 63-71.

24. Aguilera Vasquez, N. and D.E. Nielsen, *The Endocannabinoid System and Eating Behaviours: a Review of the Current State of the Evidence.* Curr Nutr Rep, 2022. **11**(4): p. 665-674.

25. McPartland, J.M., *Phylogenomic and chemotaxonomic analysis of the endocannabinoid system.* Brain Res Brain Res Rev, 2004. **45**(1): p. 18-29.

26. Lutz, B., *Neurobiology of cannabinoid receptor signaling .* Dialogues Clin Neurosci, 2020. **22**(3): p. 207-222.

27. Curioni, C. and C. Andre, *Rimonabant for overweight or obesity.* Cochrane Database Syst Rev, 2006. **2006**(4): p. CD006162.

28. Balsevich, G., et al., *Role for fatty acid amide hydrolase (FAAH) in the leptin-mediated effects on feeding and energy balance.* Proc Natl Acad Sci U S A, 2018. **115**(29): p. 7605-7610.

29. Hodges, E.L., J.P. Marshall, and N.M. Ashpole, *Age-dependent hormesis-like effects of the synthetic cannabinoid CP55940 in C57BL/6 mice.* NPJ Aging Mech Dis, 2020. **6**: p. 7.

30. Clark, T.M., et al., *Theoretical Explanation for Reduced Body Mass Index and Obesity Rates in Cannabis Users.* Cannabis Cannabinoid Res, 2018. **3**(1): p. 259-271.

31. Ben-Shabat, S., et al., *An entourage effect: inactive endogenous fatty acid glycerol esters enhance 2-arachidonoyl-glycerol cannabinoid activity.* Eur J Pharmacol, 1998. **353**(1): p. 23-31.

32. LaVigne, J.E., et al., *Cannabis sativa terpenes are cannabimimetic and selectively enhance cannabinoid activity.* Sci Rep, 2021. **11**(1): p. 8232.

33. Dvorakova, M., et al., *A Critical Evaluation of Terpenoid Signaling at Cannabinoid CB1 Receptors in a Neuronal Model.* Molecules, 2022. **27**(17).

34. Raz, N., et al., *Selected Cannabis Terpenes Synergize with Thc to Produce Increased Cb1 Receptor Activation.* Biochem Pharmacol, 2023: p. 115548.

35. Santiago, M.S., S; Arnold, JC, McGregor, IS and Connor, M, *Absence of entourage: Terpenoids commonly found in Cannabis sativa do not modulate the functional activity of Δ9-THC at human CB1 and CB2 receptors.* Preprint BioRXIV, 2019.

36. Kearn, C.S., et al., *Concurrent stimulation of cannabinoid CB1 and dopamine D2 receptors enhances heterodimer formation: a mechanism for receptor cross-talk?* Mol Pharmacol, 2005. **67**(5): p. 1697-704.

37. Ward, R.J., J.D. Pediani, and G. Milligan, *Heteromultimerization of cannabinoid CB(1) receptor and orexin OX(1) receptor generates a unique complex in which both protomers are regulated by orexin A.* J Biol Chem, 2011. **286**(43): p. 37414-28.

38. Morales, P. and P.H. Reggio, *An Update on Non-CB(1), Non-CB(2) Cannabinoid Related G-Protein-Coupled Receptors.* Cannabis Cannabinoid Res, 2017. **2**(1): p. 265-273.

39. Di Marzo, V., et al., *The role of endocannabinoids in the regulation of gastric emptying: alterations in mice fed a high-fat diet.* Br J Pharmacol, 2008. **153**(6): p. 1272-80.

40. Pazos, M.R., et al., *Cannabinoid CB1 receptors are expressed by parietal cells of the human gastric mucosa.* J Histochem Cytochem, 2008. **56**(5): p. 511-6.

41. Russo, E.B., et al., *Cannabinoid Hyperemesis Syndrome Survey and Genomic Investigation.* Cannabis Cannabinoid Res, 2022. **7**(3): p. 336-344.

42. Wallace, M.S., et al., *A Secondary Analysis from a Randomized Trial on the Effect of Plasma Tetrahydrocannabinol Levels on Pain Reduction in Painful Diabetic Peripheral Neuropathy.* J Pain, 2020. **21**(11-12): p. 1175-1186.

43. Bortolotti, M. and S. Porta, *Effect of red pepper on symptoms of irritable bowel syndrome: preliminary study.* Dig Dis Sci, 2011. **56**(11): p. 3288-95.

44. Wouters, M.M., et al., *Histamine Receptor H1-Mediated Sensitization of TRPV1 Mediates Visceral Hypersensitivity and Symptoms in Patients With Irritable Bowel Syndrome.* Gastroenterology, 2016. **150**(4): p. 875-87 e9.

45. Coates, M.D., et al., *Symptoms and Extraintestinal Manifestations in Active Cannabis Users with Inflammatory Bowel Disease.* Cannabis Cannabinoid Res, 2022. **7**(4): p. 445-450.

46. Pertwee, R.G., *The diverse CB1 and CB2 receptor pharmacology of three plant cannabinoids: delta9-tetrahydrocannabinol, cannabidiol and delta9-tetrahydro-cannabivarin*. Br J Pharmacol, 2008. **153**(2): p. 199-215.

47. Walter, L. and N. Stella, *Cannabinoids and neuroinflammation*. Br J Pharmacol, 2004. **141**(5): p. 775-85.

48. , Votrubec, C., et al., *Cannabinoid therapeutics in orofacial pain management: a systematic review*. Aust Dent J, 2022. **67**(4): p. 314-327.

49. Villanueva, M.R.B., et al., *Efficacy, Safety, and Regulation of Cannabidiol on Chronic Pain: A Systematic Review*. Cureus, 2022. **14**(7): p. e26913.

50. Monteleone, P., et al., *Blood levels of the endocannabinoid anandamide are increased in anorexia nervosa and in binge-eating disorder, but not in bulimia nervosa*. Neuropsychopharmacology, 2005. **30**(6): p. 1216-21.

51. Peck, S.K., et al., *Psilocybin therapy for females with anorexia nervosa: a phase 1, open-label feasibility study*. Nat Med, 2023.

52. Cawthorne MA, W.E., Zaibi M, Stott C, Wright S. *The CB-1 antagonist, delta-9-tetrahydrocannabivarin (THCV) has anti-obesity activity in dietary-induced obese (DIO) mice*. in *International Cannabinoid Research Society,*. 2007. Burlington, Vermont, USA.

53. Sexton, M., et al., *The Management of Cancer Symptoms and Treatment-Induced Side Effects With Cannabis or Cannabinoids*. J Natl Cancer Inst Monogr, 2021. **2021**(58): p. 86-98.

54. Jatoi, A., et al., *Dronabinol versus megestrol acetate versus combination therapy for cancer-associated anorexia: a North Central Cancer Treatment Group study*. J Clin Oncol, 2002. **20**(2): p. 567-73.

55. Kalant, H., *Medicinal use of cannabis: history and current status*. Pain Res Manag, 2001. **6**(2): p. 80-91.

56. Rousseaux, C., et al., *Lactobacillus acidophilus modulates intestinal pain and induces opioid and cannabinoid receptors*. Nat Med, 2007. **13**(1): p. 35-7.

57. Everard, A., et al., *Cross-talk between Akkermansia muciniphila and intestinal epithelium controls diet-induced obesity*. Proc Natl Acad Sci U S A, 2013. **110**(22): p. 9066-71.

58. Cuddihey, H., W.K. MacNaughton, and K.A. Sharkey, *Role of the Endocannabinoid System in the Regulation of Intestinal Homeostasis*. Cell Mol Gastroenterol Hepatol, 2022. **14**(4): p. 947-963.

59. Srivastava, R.K., B. Lutz, and I. Ruiz de Azua, *The Microbiome and Gut Endocannabinoid System in the Regulation of Stress Responses and Metabolism*. Front Cell Neurosci, 2022. **16**: p. 867267.

60. Goel, A., C.R. Boland, and D.P. Chauhan, *Specific inhibition of cyclooxygenase-2 (COX-2) expression by dietary curcumin in HT-29 human colon cancer cells*. Cancer Lett, 2001. **172**(2): p. 111-8.

61. Ring, J., et al., *Antihistamines in urticaria*. Clin Exp Allergy, 1999. **29 Suppl 1**: p. 31-7.

62. Alam, S.B., et al., *Quercetin and Resveratrol Differentially Decrease Expression of the High-Affinity IgE Receptor (FcepsilonRI) by Human and Mouse Mast Cells.* Molecules, 2022. **27**(19).

63. Koch, M., et al., *Rhythmic control of endocannabinoids in the rat pineal gland.* Chronobiol Int, 2015. **32**(6): p. 869-74.

64. Rijo-Ferreira, F. and J.S. Takahashi, *Genomics of circadian rhythms in health and disease.* Genome Med, 2019. **11**(1): p. 82.

65. Iliff, J.J., et al., *A paravascular pathway facilitates CSF flow through the brain parenchyma and the clearance of interstitial solutes, including amyloid beta.* Sci Transl Med, 2012. **4**(147): p. 147ra111.

66. Murillo-Rodriguez, E., et al., *The Endocannabinoid System Modulating Levels of Consciousness, Emotions and Likely Dream Contents.* CNS Neurol Disord Drug Targets, 2017. **16**(4): p. 370-379.

67. Vaughn, L.K., et al., *Endocannabinoid signalling: has it got rhythm?* Br J Pharmacol, 2010. **160**(3): p. 530-43.

68. Hanlon, E.C., et al., *Sleep Restriction Enhances the Daily Rhythm of Circulating Levels of Endocannabinoid 2-Arachidonoylglycerol.* Sleep, 2016. **39**(3): p. 653-64.

69. Santucci, V., et al., *Arousal-enhancing properties of the CB1 cannabinoid receptor antagonist SR 141716A in rats as assessed by electroencephalographic spectral and sleep-waking cycle analysis.* Life Sci, 1996. **58**(6): p. PL103-10.

70. Suraev, A.S., McGregor, I; Marshall, N; Kao, T; D/Rozario, A, Grunstein, R, Hoyos, C. *Acute Effects of Cannabinoids in Insomnia Disorder, A Randomized, Placebo-controlled Trial Using High Density EEG. in International Cannabinoid Research Society.* 2023. Canada.

71. Lissoni, P., et al., *Effects of tetrahydrocannabinol on melatonin secretion in man.* Horm Metab Res, 1986. **18**(1): p. 77-8.

72. Sexton, M., et al., *Evaluation of Cannabinoid and Terpenoid Content: Cannabis Flower Compared to Supercritical CO2 Concentrate.* Planta Med, 2018. **84**(4): p. 234-241.

73. Vigil, J.M., et al., *Systematic combinations of major cannabinoid and terpene contents in Cannabis flower and patient outcomes: a proof-of-concept assessment of the Vigil Index of Cannabis Chemovars.* J Cannabis Res, 2023. **5**(1): p. 4.

74. Elzinga S, Fischedick J, Podkolinski R and Raber JC, *Cannabinoids and Terpenes as Chemotaxonomic Markers in Cannabis.* Natural Products Chemistry and Research, 2015. **3**(4).

75. Kaul, M., P.C. Zee, and A.S. Sahni, *Effects of Cannabinoids on Sleep and their Therapeutic Potential for Sleep Disorders.* Neurotherapeutics, 2021. **18**(1): p. 217-227.

76. Murillo-Rodriguez, E., et al., *Potential effects of cannabidiol as a wake-promoting agent.* Curr Neuropharmacol, 2014. **12**(3): p. 269-72.

77. Wang, M.F., M, Abbott, S, Patel, V, Chang, E, Clark JO, Stella, N, Mucowski PJ, *A Cannabidiol/Terpene Formulation That Increases Restorative Sleep in Insomniacs: A Double-Blind, Placebo-controlled, Randomized, Crossover Pilot Study.* MedRxIV, 2023.

78. Corroon, J., *Cannabinol and Sleep: Separating Fact from Fiction.* Cannabis Cannabinoid Res, 2021. **6**(5): p. 366-371.

79. Pivik, R.T., et al., *Delta-9-tetrahydrocannabinol and synhexl: effects on human sleep patterns.* Clin Pharmacol Ther, 1972. **13**(3): p. 426-35.

80. Feinberg, I., et al., *Effects of marijuana extract and tetrahydrocannabinol on electroencephalographic sleep patterns.* Clin Pharmacol Ther, 1976. **19**(6): p. 782-94.

81. Campbell, L.M., et al., *Cannabis use is associated with greater total sleep time in middle-aged and older adults with and without HIV: A preliminary report utilizing digital health technologies.* Cannabis, 2020. **3**(2): p. 180-189.

82. Nowakowski, S., J. Meers, and E. Heimbach, *Sleep and Women's Health.* Sleep Med Res, 2013. **4**(1): p. 1-22.

83. Di Blasio, A.M., M. Vignali, and D. Gentilini, *The endocannabinoid pathway and the female reproductive organs.* J Mol Endocrinol, 2013. **50**(1): p. R1-9.

84. Maccarrone, M., et al., *Low fatty acid amide hydrolase and high anandamide levels are associated with failure to achieve an ongoing pregnancy after IVF and embryo transfer.* Mol Hum Reprod, 2002. **8**(2): p. 188-95.

85. Cui, N., et al., *The correlation of anandamide with gonadotrophin and sex steroid hormones during the menstrual cycle.* Iran J Basic Med Sci, 2017. **20**(11): p. 1268-1274.

86. Habayeb, O.M., et al., *Plasma levels of the endocannabinoid anandamide in women--a potential role in pregnancy maintenance and labor?* J Clin Endocrinol Metab, 2004. **89**(11): p. 5482-7.

87. El-Talatini, M.R., A.H. Taylor, and J.C. Konje, *The relationship between plasma levels of the endocannabinoid, anandamide, sex steroids, and gonadotrophins during the menstrual cycle.* Fertil Steril, 2010. **93**(6): p. 1989-96.

88. Nallendran, V., et al., *The plasma levels of the endocannabinoid, anandamide, increase with the induction of labour.* BJOG, 2010. **117**(7): p. 863-9.

89. Yin, W., et al., *Melatonin for premenstrual syndrome: A potential remedy but not ready.* Front Endocrinol (Lausanne), 2022. **13**: p. 1084249.

90. Baker, F.C. and K.A. Lee, *Menstrual Cycle Effects on Sleep.* Sleep Med Clin, 2018. **13**(3): p. 283-294.

91. Sciarra, F., et al., *Disruption of Circadian Rhythms: A Crucial Factor in the Etiology of Infertility.* Int J Mol Sci, 2020. **21**(11).

92. Hurd, Y.L., et al., *Cannabis and the Developing Brain: Insights into Its Long-Lasting Effects.* J Neurosci, 2019. **39**(42): p. 8250-8258.

93. Lo, J.O., et al., *Cannabis Use in Pregnancy and Neonatal Outcomes: A Systematic Review and Meta-Analysis.* Cannabis Cannabinoid Res, 2023.

94. de Almeida, C.M.O., et al., *The Effect of Cannabidiol for Restless Legs Syndrome/ Willis-Ekbom Disease in Parkinson's Disease Patients with REM Sleep Behavior Disorder: A Post Hoc Exploratory Analysis of Phase 2/3 Clinical Trial.* Cannabis Cannabinoid Res, 2023. **8**(2): p. 374-378.

95. Farabi, S.S., et al., *Impact of dronabinol on quantitative electroencephalogram (qEEG) measures of sleep in obstructive sleep apnea syndrome.* J Clin Sleep Med, 2014. **10**(1): p. 49-56.

96. Carley, D.W., et al., *Pharmacotherapy of Apnea by Cannabimimetic Enhancement, the PACE Clinical Trial: Effects of Dronabinol in Obstructive Sleep Apnea.* Sleep, 2018. **41**(1).

97. Sznitman, S.R., et al., *Posttraumatic stress disorder, sleep and medical cannabis treatment: A daily diary study.* J Anxiety Disord, 2022. **92**: p. 102632.

98. Fuss, J., et al., *Masturbation to Orgasm Stimulates the Release of the Endocannabinoid 2-Arachidonoylglycerol in Humans.* J Sex Med, 2017. **14**(11): p. 1372-1379.

99. Piomelli, D. and E.B. Russo, *The Cannabis sativa Versus Cannabis indica Debate: An Interview with Ethan Russo, MD.* Cannabis Cannabinoid Res, 2016. **1**(1): p. 44-46.

100. Johnson, M.B., et al., *The Effects of beta-myrcene on Simulated Driving and Divided Attention: A Double-Blind, Placebo-Controlled, Crossover Pilot Study.* Cannabis, 2023. **6**(1): p. 9-19.

101. Meloni, M., et al., *Preliminary finding of a randomized, double-blind, placebo-controlled, crossover study to evaluate the safety and efficacy of 5-hydroxytryptophan on REM sleep behavior disorder in Parkinson's disease.* Sleep Breath, 2022. **26**(3): p. 1023-1031.

102. Bruni, O., et al., *L -5-Hydroxytryptophan treatment of sleep terrors in children.* Eur J Pediatr, 2004. **163**(7): p. 402-7.

103. Sexton, M., et al., *A Cross-Sectional Survey of Medical Cannabis Users: Patterns of Use and Perceived Efficacy.* Cannabis Cannabinoid Res, 2016. **1**(1): p. 131-138.

104. Corroon, J.M., Jr., L.K. Mischley, and M. Sexton, *Cannabis as a substitute for prescription drugs - a cross-sectional study.* J Pain Res, 2017. **10**: p. 989-998.

105. Cuttler, C., A. Spradlin, and R.J. McLaughlin, *A naturalistic examination of the perceived effects of cannabis on negative affect.* J Affect Disord, 2018. **235**: p. 198-205.

106. Childs, E., J.A. Lutz, and H. de Wit, *Dose-related effects of delta-9-THC on emotional responses to acute psychosocial stress.* Drug Alcohol Depend, 2017. **177**: p. 136-144.

107. Hunault, C.C., et al., *Acute subjective effects after smoking joints containing up to 69 mg Delta9-tetrahydrocannabinol in recreational users: a randomized, crossover clinical trial.* Psychopharmacology (Berl), 2014. **231**(24): p. 4723-33.

108. Viveros, M.P., E.M. Marco, and S.E. File, *Endocannabinoid system and stress and anxiety responses.* Pharmacol Biochem Behav, 2005. **81**(2): p. 331-42.

109. Milanos, S., et al., *Metabolic Products of Linalool and Modulation of GABA(A) Receptors.* Front Chem, 2017. **5**: p. 46.

110. Gulluni, N., et al., *Cannabis Essential Oil: A Preliminary Study for the Evaluation of the Brain Effects.* Evid Based Complement Alternat Med, 2018. **2018**: p. 1709182.

111. Bahi, A., et al., *beta-Caryophyllene, a CB2 receptor agonist produces multiple behavioral changes relevant to anxiety and depression in mice.* Physiol Behav, 2014. **135**: p. 119-24.

112. Chouker, A., et al., *Motion sickness, stress and the endocannabinoid system.* PLoS One, 2010. **5**(5): p. e10752.

113. Hill, M.N. and J.G. Tasker, *Endocannabinoid signaling, glucocorticoid-mediated negative feedback, and regulation of the hypothalamic-pituitary-adrenal axis.* Neuroscience, 2012. **204**: p. 5-16.

114. Patel, S., et al., *Endocannabinoid signaling negatively modulates stress-induced activation of the hypothalamic-pituitary-adrenal axis.* Endocrinology, 2004. **145**(12): p. 5431-8.

115. McEwen, B.S., *Stress, adaptation, and disease. Allostasis and allostatic load.* Ann N Y Acad Sci, 1998. **840**: p. 33-44.

116. Sharp, P.B., et al., *Mindfulness training induces structural connectome changes in insula networks.* Sci Rep, 2018. **8**(1): p. 7929.

117. Blest-Hopley, G., V. Giampietro, and S. Bhattacharyya, *Regular cannabis use is associated with altered activation of central executive and default mode networks even after prolonged abstinence in adolescent users: Results from a complementary meta-analysis.* Neurosci Biobehav Rev, 2019. **96**: p. 45-55.

118. Vigil, J.M., S.S. Stith, and T. Chanel, *Cannabis consumption and prosociality.* Sci Rep, 2022. **12**(1): p. 8352.

119. Wang, D., et al., *Neural substrates underlying the effects of oxytocin: a quantitative meta-analysis of pharmaco-imaging studies.* Soc Cogn Affect Neurosci, 2017. **12**(10): p. 1565-1573.

120. LaSalle, J.M., *Placenta keeps the score of maternal cannabis use and child anxiety.* Proc Natl Acad Sci U S A, 2021. **118**(47).

121. O'Connell, C.M. and P.A. Fried, *Prenatal exposure to cannabis: a preliminary report of postnatal consequences in school-age children.* Neurotoxicol Teratol, 1991. **13**(6): p. 631-9.

122. Goldschmidt, L., N.L. Day, and G.A. Richardson, *Effects of prenatal marijuana exposure on child behavior problems at age 10.* Neurotoxicol Teratol, 2000. **22**(3): p. 325-36.

123. Rompala, G., Y. Nomura, and Y.L. Hurd, *Maternal cannabis use is associated with suppression of immune gene networks in placenta and increased anxiety phenotypes in offspring.* Proc Natl Acad Sci U S A, 2021. **118**(47).

124. He, Q., et al., *Risk of Dementia in Long-Term Benzodiazepine Users: Evidence from a Meta-Analysis of Observational Studies.* J Clin Neurol, 2019. **15**(1): p. 9-19.

125. Bansal, N., et al., *Antidepressant use and risk of adverse outcomes: population-based cohort study.* BJPsych Open, 2022. **8**(5): p. e164.

126. Moncrieff, J., et al., *The serotonin theory of depression: a systematic umbrella review of the evidence.* Mol Psychiatry, 2022.

127. Danhauer, S.C., et al., *Long-Term Effects of Cognitive-Behavioral Therapy and Yoga for Worried Older Adults.* Am J Geriatr Psychiatry, 2022. **30**(9): p. 979-990.

128. Zanardi, R., et al., *Add-On Treatment with Passiflora incarnata L., herba, during Benzodiazepine Tapering in Patients with Depression and Anxiety: A Real-World Study.* Pharmaceuticals (Basel), 2023. **16**(3).

129. Sakalem, M.E., et al., *Behavioral Pharmacology of Five Uncommon Passiflora Species Indicates Sedative and Anxiolytic-like Potential.* Cent Nerv Syst Agents Med Chem, 2022. **22**(2): p. 125-138.

130. Awad, R., et al., *Phytochemical and biological analysis of skullcap (Scutellaria lateriflora L.): a medicinal plant with anxiolytic properties.* Phytomedicine, 2003. **10**(8): p. 640-9.

131. Zhang, W., et al., *Medicinal herbs for the treatment of anxiety: A systematic review and network meta-analysis.* Pharmacol Res, 2022. **179**: p. 106204.

132. Pohjanvirta, R. and A. Nasri, *The Potent Phytoestrogen 8-Prenylnaringenin: A Friend or a Foe?* Int J Mol Sci, 2022. **23**(6).

133. Soma, R., et al., *Effect of glycyrrhizin on cortisol metabolism in humans.* Endocr Regul, 1994. **28**(1): p. 31-4.

134. Schellenberg, R., *Treatment for the premenstrual syndrome with agnus castus fruit extract: prospective, randomised, placebo controlled study.* BMJ, 2001. **322**(7279): p. 134-7.

135. Nicolussi, S., et al., *Guineensine is a novel inhibitor of endocannabinoid uptake showing cannabimimetic behavioral effects in BALB/c mice.* Pharmacol Res, 2014. **80**: p. 52-65.

136. Pacher, P. and G. Kunos, *Modulating the endocannabinoid system in human health and disease--successes and failures.* FEBS J, 2013. **280**(9): p. 1918-43.

137. Koren, T. and A. Rolls, *Immunoception: Defining brain-regulated immunity.* Neuron, 2022. **110**(21): p. 3425-3428.

138. Marcu, J.P., et al., *Cannabidiol enhances the inhibitory effects of delta9-tetrahydrocannabinol on human glioblastoma cell proliferation and survival.* Mol Cancer Ther, 2010. **9**(1): p. 180-9.

139. Vallee, M., et al., *Pregnenolone can protect the brain from cannabis intoxication.* Science, 2014. **343**(6166): p. 94-8.

140. Turcotte, C., et al., *The CB2 receptor and its role as a regulator of inflammation.* Cell Mol Life Sci, 2016. **73**(23): p. 4449-4470.

141. Sexton, M., et al., *Cannabis use by individuals with multiple sclerosis: effects on specific immune parameters.* Inflammopharmacology, 2014. **22**(5): p. 295-303.

142. Sexton, M.S., A; Moller, T; Stella, N., *Differential migratory properties of monocytes isolated from human subjects naive and non-naive to Cannabis.* Inflammopharmacology, 2012. **April 11.**

143. Sexton, M., et al., *Differential migratory properties of monocytes isolated from human subjects naive and non-naive to Cannabis.* Inflammopharmacology, 2013. **21**(3): p. 253-9.

144. Carnevale, D., *Neuroimmune axis of cardiovascular control: mechanisms and therapeutic implications.* Nat Rev Cardiol, 2022. **19**(6): p. 379-394.

145. Jessen, N.A., et al., *The Glymphatic System: A Beginner's Guide.* Neurochem Res, 2015. **40**(12): p. 2583-99.

146. Mogensen, F.L., C. Delle, and M. Nedergaard, *The Glymphatic System (En)during Inflammation.* Int J Mol Sci, 2021. **22**(14).

147. Ellis, R.J., et al., *Recent cannabis use in HIV is associated with reduced inflammatory markers in CSF and blood.* Neurol Neuroimmunol Neuroinflamm, 2020. **7**(5).

148. Ellis, R.J., et al., *Beneficial Effects of Cannabis on Blood-Brain Barrier Function in Human Immunodeficiency Virus.* Clin Infect Dis, 2021. **73**(1): p. 124-129.

149. Shanley, J.E., et al., *Longitudinal evaluation of neurologic-post acute sequelae SARS-CoV-2 infection symptoms.* Ann Clin Transl Neurol, 2022. **9**(7): p. 995-1010.

150. Park, Y.M., T. Shekhtman, and J.R. Kelsoe, *Effect of the Type and Number of Adverse Childhood Experiences and the Timing of Adverse Experiences on Clinical Outcomes in Individuals with Bipolar Disorder.* Brain Sci, 2020. **10**(5).

151. Eisenstein, T.K., et al., *Anandamide and Delta9-tetrahydrocannabinol directly inhibit cells of the immune system via CB2 receptors.* J Neuroimmunol, 2007. **189**(1-2): p. 17-22.

152. Baczynsky, W.O. and A.M. Zimmerman, *Effects of delta 9-tetrahydrocannabinol, cannabinol and cannabidiol on the immune system in mice. II. In vitro investigation using cultured mouse splenocytes.* Pharmacology, 1983. **26**(1): p. 12-9.

153. Maresz, K., et al., *Direct suppression of CNS autoimmune inflammation via the cannabinoid receptor CB1 on neurons and CB2 on autoreactive T cells.* Nat Med, 2007. **13**(4): p. 492-7.

154. Longoria, V., et al., *Neurological Benefits, Clinical Challenges, and Neuropathologic Promise of Medical Marijuana: A Systematic Review of Cannabinoid Effects in Multiple Sclerosis and Experimental Models of Demyelination.* Biomedicines, 2022. **10**(3).

155. Haddad, F., G. Dokmak, and R. Karaman, *The Efficacy of Cannabis on Multiple Sclerosis-Related Symptoms.* Life (Basel), 2022. **12**(5).

156. Galiegue, S., et al., *Expression of central and peripheral cannabinoid receptors in human immune tissues and leukocyte subpopulations.* Eur J Biochem, 1995. **232**(1): p. 54-61.

157. Wiese, B.M., et al., *The endocannabinoid system and breathing.* Front Neurosci, 2023. **17**: p. 1126004.

158. Morgan, N., et al., *The effects of mind-body therapies on the immune system: meta-analysis.* PLoS One, 2014. **9**(7): p. e100903.

159. Pozzilli, C., M. Pugliatti, and M.S.G. Paradig, *An overview of pregnancy-related issues in patients with multiple sclerosis.* Eur J Neurol, 2015. **22 Suppl 2:** p. 34-9.

160. Thippeswamy, H. and W. Davies, *A new molecular risk pathway for postpartum mood disorders: clues from steroid sulfatase-deficient individuals.* Arch Womens Ment Health, 2021. **24**(3): p. 391-401.

161. Accortt, E.E., et al., *Lower prenatal vitamin D status and postpartum depressive symptomatology in African American women: Preliminary evidence for moderation by inflammatory cytokines.* Arch Womens Ment Health, 2016. **19**(2): p. 373-83.

162. Friedrich, J., et al., *The grass isn't always greener: The effects of cannabis on embryological development.* BMC Pharmacol Toxicol, 2016. **17**(1): p. 45.

163. Hua, D.Y., et al., *Effects of cannabidiol on anandamide levels in individuals with cannabis use disorder: findings from a randomised clinical trial for the treatment of cannabis use disorder.* Transl Psychiatry, 2023. **13**(1): p. 131.

164. Stochino Loi, E., et al., *Effect of ultramicronized-palmitoylethanolamide and co-micronized palmitoylethanolamide/polydatin on chronic pelvic pain and quality of life in endometriosis patients: An open-label pilot study.* Int J Womens Health, 2019. **11:** p. 443-449.

165. Ferreira, I., et al., *Resolvins, Protectins, and Maresins: DHA-Derived Specialized Pro-Resolving Mediators, Biosynthetic Pathways, Synthetic Approaches, and Their Role in Inflammation.* Molecules, 2022. **27**(5).

166. Watkins, B.A., et al., *Circulating levels of endocannabinoids and oxylipins altered by dietary lipids in older women are likely associated with previously identified gene targets.* Biochim Biophys Acta, 2016. **1861**(11): p. 1693-1704.

167. Cordingley, D.M. and S.M. Cornish, *Omega-3 Fatty Acids for the Management of Osteoarthritis: A Narrative Review.* Nutrients, 2022. **14**(16).

168. Karas, J.A., et al., *The Antimicrobial Activity of Cannabinoids.* Antibiotics (Basel), 2020. **9**(7).

169. Gertsch, J., et al., *Beta-caryophyllene is a dietary cannabinoid.* Proc Natl Acad Sci U S A, 2008. **105**(26): p. 9099-104.

170. Kumar, A., et al., *Cannabimimetic plants: are they new cannabinoidergic modulators?* Planta, 2019. **249**(6): p. 1681-1694.

171. Gertsch, J., *Cannabimimetic phytochemicals in the diet - an evolutionary link to food selection and metabolic stress adaptation?* Br J Pharmacol, 2017. **174**(11): p. 1464-1483.

172. Russo, E.B., et al., *Survey of Patients Employing Cannabigerol-Predominant Cannabis Preparations: Perceived Medical Effects, Adverse Events, and Withdrawal Symptoms.* Cannabis Cannabinoid Res, 2022. **7**(5): p. 706-716.

173. Chebet, J.J., et al., *Effect of d-limonene and its derivatives on breast cancer in human trials: a scoping review and narrative synthesis.* BMC Cancer, 2021. **21**(1): p. 902.

174. Fischedick, J.T., *Identification of Terpenoid Chemotypes Among High (-)-trans-Delta(9)- Tetrahydrocannabinol-Producing Cannabis sativa L. Cultivars.* Cannabis Cannabinoid Res, 2017. **2**(1): p. 34-47.

175. Guggenheim, A.G., K.M. Wright, and H.L. Zwickey, *Immune Modulation From Five Major Mushrooms: Application to Integrative Oncology.* Integr Med (Encinitas), 2014. **13**(1): p. 32-44.

176. van Breemen, R.B., Y. Tao, and W. Li, *Cyclooxygenase-2 inhibitors in ginger (Zingiber officinale).* Fitoterapia, 2011. **82**(1): p. 38-43.

177. Woelkart, K., et al., *Bioavailability and pharmacokinetics of alkamides from the roots of Echinacea angustifolia in humans.* J Clin Pharmacol, 2005. **45**(6): p. 683-9.

178. Hudson, J.B., *Applications of the phytomedicine Echinacea purpurea (Purple Coneflower) in infectious diseases.* J Biomed Biotechnol, 2012. **2012**: p. 769896.

179. Raduner, S., et al., *Alkylamides from Echinacea are a new class of cannabinomimetics. Cannabinoid type 2 receptor-dependent and -independent immunomodulatory effects.* J Biol Chem, 2006. **281**(20): p. 14192-206.

180. Anand, U., et al., *Cannabinoid receptor CB2 localisation and agonist-mediated inhibition of capsaicin responses in human sensory neurons.* Pain, 2008. **138**(3): p. 667-80.

181. Lopresti, A.L. and S.J. Smith, *An investigation into the anxiety-relieving and mood-enhancing effects of Echinacea angustifolia (EP107): A randomised, double-blind, placebo-controlled study.* J Affect Disord, 2021. **293**: p. 229-237.

182. Liu, R., et al., *Biochemometric Analysis of Fatty Acid Amide Hydrolase Inhibition by Echinacea Root Extracts.* Planta Med, 2021. **87**(4): p. 294-304.

183. Ligresti, A., et al., *Kavalactones and the endocannabinoid system: the plant-derived yangonin is a novel CB(1) receptor ligand.* Pharmacol Res, 2012. **66**(2): p. 163-9.

184. Luca, S.V., et al., *Insights into the Phytochemical and Multifunctional Biological Profile of Spices from the Genus Piper.* Antioxidants (Basel), 2021. **10**(10).

185. Korte, G., et al., *An examination of anthocyanins' and anthocyanidins' affinity for cannabinoid receptors.* J Med Food, 2009. **12**(6): p. 1407-10.

186. Gertsch, J., *Anti-inflammatory cannabinoids in diet: Towards a better understanding of CB(2) receptor action?* Commun Integr Biol, 2008. **1**(1): p. 26-8.

187. Ashton, J.C. and M. Glass, *The cannabinoid CB2 receptor as a target for inflammation-dependent neurodegeneration.* Curr Neuropharmacol, 2007. **5**(2): p. 73-80.

188. Klauke, A.L., et al., *The cannabinoid CB(2) receptor-selective phytocannabinoid beta-caryophyllene exerts analgesic effects in mouse models of inflammatory and neuropathic pain.* Eur Neuropsychopharmacol, 2014. **24**(4): p. 608-20.

189. Frisoni, G.B., et al., *The clinical use of structural MRI in Alzheimer disease.* Nat Rev Neurol, 2010. **6**(2): p. 67-77.

190. Little, P.J., et al., *Pharmacology and stereoselectivity of structurally novel cannabinoids in mice.* J Pharmacol Exp Ther, 1988. **247**(3): p. 1046-51.

191. Walmsley, B., F.J. Alvarez, and R.E. Fyffe, *Diversity of structure and function at mammalian central synapses.* Trends Neurosci, 1998. **21**(2): p. 81-8.

192. Callen, L., et al., *Cannabinoid receptors CB1 and CB2 form functional heteromers in brain.* J Biol Chem, 2012. **287**(25): p. 20851-65.

193. Varvel, S.A., et al., *Fatty acid amide hydrolase (-/-) mice exhibit an increased sensitivity to the disruptive effects of anandamide or oleamide in a working memory water maze task.* J Pharmacol Exp Ther, 2006. **317**(1): p. 251-7.

194. Adam, K.C.S., et al., *Delta(9)-Tetrahydrocannabinol (THC) impairs visual working memory performance: a randomized crossover trial.* Neuropsychopharmacology, 2020. **45**(11): p. 1807-1816.

195. Eyo, U.B., et al., *Microglia provide structural resolution to injured dendrites after severe seizures.* Cell Rep, 2021. **35**(5): p. 109080.

196. Glass, M., M. Dragunow, and R.L. Faull, *Cannabinoid receptors in the human brain: a detailed anatomical and quantitative autoradiographic study in the fetal, neonatal and adult human brain.* Neuroscience, 1997. **77**(2): p. 299-318.

197. Hartley, C., Phelps, EA, *Extinction Learning*, in *Encyclopedia of the Sciences of Learning*, N. Seel, Editor. 2012, Springer: Boston, MA.

198. Marsicano, G., et al., *The endogenous cannabinoid system controls extinction of aversive memories.* Nature, 2002. **418**(6897): p. 530-4.

199. Hill, M.N., et al., *Reductions in circulating endocannabinoid levels in individuals with post-traumatic stress disorder following exposure to the World Trade Center attacks.* Psychoneuroendocrinology, 2013. **38**(12): p. 2952-61.

200. Bluett, R.J., et al., *Endocannabinoid signalling modulates susceptibility to traumatic stress exposure.* Nat Commun, 2017. **8**: p. 14782.

201. Mayo, L.M., et al., *Elevated Anandamide, Enhanced Recall of Fear Extinction, and Attenuated Stress Responses Following Inhibition of Fatty Acid Amide Hydrolase: A Randomized, Controlled Experimental Medicine Trial.* Biol Psychiatry, 2020. **87**(6): p. 538-547.

202. Song, C., et al., *Bidirectional Effects of Cannabidiol on Contextual Fear Memory Extinction.* Front Pharmacol, 2016. **7**: p. 493.

203. Bonn-Miller, M.O., et al., *The short-term impact of 3 smoked cannabis preparations versus placebo on PTSD symptoms: A randomized cross-over clinical trial.* PLoS One, 2021. **16**(3): p. e0246990.

204. Shao, L.X., et al., *Psilocybin induces rapid and persistent growth of dendritic spines in frontal cortex in vivo.* Neuron, 2021. **109**(16): p. 2535-2544 e4.

205. Mitchell, J.M., et al., *MDMA-assisted therapy for severe PTSD: a randomized, double-blind, placebo-controlled phase 3 study.* Nat Med, 2021. **27**(6): p. 1025-1033.

206. Pacheco, D.D.F., T.R.L. Romero, and I.D.G. Duarte, *Ketamine induces central antinociception mediated by endogenous cannabinoids and activation of CB(1) receptors.* Neurosci Lett, 2019. **699**: p. 140-144.

207. Ferreira, R.C.M., et al., *The Involvement of the Endocannabinoid System in the Peripheral Antinociceptive Action of Ketamine.* J Pain, 2018. **19**(5): p. 487-495.

208. Ibarra-Lecue, I., et al., *Chronic cannabis promotes pro-hallucinogenic signaling of 5-HT2A receptors through Akt/mTOR pathway.* Neuropsychopharmacology, 2018. **43**(10): p. 2028-2035.

209. Fagundo, A.B., et al., *Modulation of the Endocannabinoids N-Arachidonoyletha-nolamine (AEA) and 2-Arachidonoylglycerol (2-AG) on Executive Functions in Humans.* PLoS One, 2013. **8**(6): p. e66387.

210. Hill, M.N., et al., *Alterations in behavioral flexibility by cannabinoid CB1 receptor agonists and antagonists.* Psychopharmacology (Berl), 2006. **187**(2): p. 245-59.

211. de Manzano, O., et al., *Thinking outside a less intact box: thalamic dopamine D2 receptor densities are negatively related to psychometric creativity in healthy individuals.* PLoS One, 2010. **5**(5): p. e10670.

212. Howes, O.D., et al., *The nature of dopamine dysfunction in schizophrenia and what this means for treatment.* Arch Gen Psychiatry, 2012. **69**(8): p. 776-86.

213. Hirvonen, J., et al., *Reversible and regionally selective downregulation of brain cannabinoid CB1 receptors in chronic daily cannabis smokers.* Mol Psychiatry, 2012. **17**(6): p. 642-9.

214. Ceccarini, J., et al., *[18F]MK-9470 PET measurement of cannabinoid CB1 receptor availability in chronic cannabis users.* Addict Biol, 2015. **20**(2): p. 357-67.

215. D'Souza, D.C., et al., *Rapid Changes in Cannabinoid 1 Receptor Availability in Cannabis-Dependent Male Subjects After Abstinence From Cannabis.* Biol Psychiatry Cogn Neurosci Neuroimaging, 2016. **1**(1): p. 60-67.

216. Bhattacharyya, S., et al., *Induction of psychosis by Delta9-tetrahydrocannabinol reflects modulation of prefrontal and striatal function during attentional salience processing.* Arch Gen Psychiatry, 2012. **69**(1): p. 27-36.

217. Bossong, M.G., et al., *Default mode network in the effects of Delta9-Tetrahydrocan-nabinol (THC) on human executive function.* PLoS One, 2013. **8**(7): p. e70074.

218. Karhson, D.S., et al., *Plasma anandamide concentrations are lower in children with autism spectrum disorder.* Mol Autism, 2018. **9**: p. 18.

219. Mottron, L., et al., *Sex differences in brain plasticity: a new hypothesis for sex ratio bias in autism.* Mol Autism, 2015. **6**: p. 33.

220. Cavalier-Smith, T., *Origin of mitochondria by intracellular enslavement of a photo-synthetic purple bacterium.* Proc Biol Sci, 2006. **273**(1596): p. 1943-52.

221. Benard, G., et al., *Mitochondrial CB(1) receptors regulate neuronal energy metabolism.* Nat Neurosci, 2012. **15**(4): p. 558-64.

222. Harte-Hargrove, L.C., N.J. Maclusky, and H.E. Scharfman, *Brain-derived neurotrophic factor-estrogen interactions in the hippocampal mossy fiber pathway: implications for normal brain function and disease.* Neuroscience, 2013. **239**: p. 46-66.

223. van de Pol, L.A., et al., *Hippocampal atrophy in Alzheimer disease: age matters.* Neurology, 2006. **66**(2): p. 236-8.

224. Sienski, G., et al., *APOE4 disrupts intracellular lipid homeostasis in human iP-SC-derived glia.* Sci Transl Med, 2021. **13**(583).

225. Currais, A., et al., *Amyloid proteotoxicity initiates an inflammatory response blocked by cannabinoids.* NPJ Aging Mech Dis, 2016. **2**: p. 16012.

226. Huss, R., *Feminine Forever.* Journal of the American Medical Association, 1966. **197**(2): p. 156.

227. Woodruff, J.D. and J.H. Pickar, *Incidence of endometrial hyperplasia in postmenopausal women taking conjugated estrogens (Premarin) with medroxyprogesterone acetate or conjugated estrogens alone. The Menopause Study Group.* Am J Obstet Gynecol, 1994. **170**(5 Pt 1): p. 1213-23.

228. Schierbeck, L.L., et al., *Effect of hormone replacement therapy on cardiovascular events in recently postmenopausal women: randomised trial.* BMJ, 2012. **345**: p. e6409.

229. Saleh, R.N.M., et al., *Hormone replacement therapy is associated with improved cognition and larger brain volumes in at-risk APOE4 women: results from the European Prevention of Alzheimer's Disease (EPAD) cohort.* Alzheimers Res Ther, 2023. **15**(1): p. 10.

230. Walker, K.L., et al., *Prevalence, Perceptions, and Patterns of Cannabis Use Among Cardiac Inpatients at a Tertiary-Care Hospital: A Cross-Sectional Survey.* CJC Open, 2023. **5**(4): p. 315-324.

231. Corroon, J., et al., *Trends in Cannabis Use, Blood Pressure and Hypertension in Middle-Aged Adults: Findings from NHANES, 2009-2018, Corroon, et al.* Am J Hypertens, 2023.

232. Chang, Y.H., S.T. Lee, and W.W. Lin, *Effects of cannabinoids on LPS-stimulated inflammatory mediator release from macrophages: involvement of eicosanoids.* J Cell Biochem, 2001. **81**(4): p. 715-23.

233. Dujic, G., et al., *Chronic Effects of Oral Cannabidiol Delivery on 24-h Ambulatory Blood Pressure in Patients with Hypertension (HYPER-H21-4): A Randomized, Placebo-Controlled, and Crossover Study.* Cannabis Cannabinoid Res, 2023.

234. Subramaniam, V.N., et al., *The Cardiovascular Effects of Marijuana: Are the Potential Adverse Effects Worth the High?* Mo Med, 2019. **116**(2): p. 146-153.

235. Ahmed, A., et al., *Cannabinoids in late-onset Alzheimer's disease.* Clin Pharmacol Ther, 2015. **97**(6): p. 597-606.

236. Bilkei-Gorzo, A., et al., *A chronic low dose of Delta(9)-tetrahydrocannabinol (THC) restores cognitive function in old mice.* Nat Med, 2017. **23**(6): p. 782-787.

237. Sarne, Y., et al., *Reversal of age-related cognitive impairments in mice by an extremely low dose of tetrahydrocannabinol.* Neurobiol Aging, 2018. **61**: p. 177-186.

238. Xiao, Y., et al., *Tetrahydrocurcumin ameliorates Alzheimer's pathological phenotypes by inhibition of microglial cell cycle arrest and apoptosis via Ras/ERK signaling.* Biomed Pharmacother, 2021. **139**: p. 111651.

239. Wang, Z., et al., *Cannabidiol induces autophagy and improves neuronal health associated with SIRT1 mediated longevity.* Geroscience, 2022. **44**(3): p. 1505-1524.

240. Notaras, M. and M. van den Buuse, *Neurobiology of BDNF in fear memory, sensitivity to stress, and stress-related disorders.* Mol Psychiatry, 2020. **25**(10): p. 2251-2274.

241. Shi, Y., et al., *Long-term diazepam treatment enhances microglial spine engulfment and impairs cognitive performance via the mitochondrial 18 kDa translocator protein (TSPO).* Nat Neurosci, 2022. **25**(3): p. 317-329.

242. Dave, N., et al., *Dietary choline intake is necessary to prevent systems-wide organ pathology and reduce Alzheimer's disease hallmarks.* Aging Cell, 2023. **22**(2): p. e13775.

243. Hou, L., et al., *Lifetime Cumulative Effect of Reproductive Factors on Stroke and Its Subtypes in Postmenopausal Chinese Women: A Prospective Cohort Study.* Neurology, 2023. **100**(15): p. e1574-e1586.

244. Jeon, Y.J., et al., *Attenuation of inducible nitric oxide synthase gene expression by delta 9-tetrahydrocannabinol is mediated through the inhibition of nuclear factor-kappa B/Rel activation.* Mol Pharmacol, 1996. **50**(2): p. 334-41.

245. Coetzee, C., et al., *Anticoagulant effects of a Cannabis extract in an obese rat model.* Phytomedicine, 2007. **14**(5): p. 333-7.

246. Hampson, A.A., J, Grimaldi, M, *Cannabinoids as Antioxidants and Neuroprotectants,* U.D.o.H.A.H. Services, Editor. 1999: United States.

247. Garberg, H.T., et al., *Short-term effects of cannabidiol after global hypoxia-ischemia in newborn piglets.* Pediatr Res, 2016. **80**(5): p. 710-718.

248. Mori, M.A., et al., *Cannabidiol reduces neuroinflammation and promotes neuroplasticity and functional recovery after brain ischemia.* Prog Neuropsychopharmacol Biol Psychiatry, 2017. **75**: p. 94-105.

249. Henry, N., et al., *Cannabidiol's Multifactorial Mechanisms Has Therapeutic Potential for Aneurysmal Subarachnoid Hemorrhage: a Review.* Transl Stroke Res, 2023. **14**(3): p. 283-296.

250. Kossatz, E., R. Maldonado, and P. Robledo, *CB2 cannabinoid receptors modulate HIF-1alpha and TIM-3 expression in a hypoxia-ischemia mouse model.* Eur Neuropsychopharmacol, 2016. **26**(12): p. 1972-1988.

251. Sanchez, A.M., et al., *Elevated Systemic Levels of Endocannabinoids and Related Mediators Across the Menstrual Cycle in Women With Endometriosis.* Reprod Sci, 2016. **23**(8): p. 1071-9.

252. Farlow, J.W., *On the use of belladonna and Cannabis indica by the rectum in gynecological practice.* Boston Med Surg J, 1889. **120**: p. 507-509.

253. Reynolds, J., *Therapeutical uses and toxic effects of Cannabis indica.* Lancet, 1868. **1**: p. 637-638.

254. Solis-Cohen, S., and T.S. Githens., *Pharmacotherapeutics, materia medica and drug action,* 1928, D. Appleton: New York.

255. Carrubba, A.R., et al., *Use of Cannabis for Self-Management of Chronic Pelvic Pain.* J Womens Health (Larchmt), 2021. **30**(9): p. 1344-1351.

256. Akerman, S., P.R. Holland, and P.J. Goadsby, *Cannabinoid (CB1) receptor activation inhibits trigeminovascular neurons.* J Pharmacol Exp Ther, 2007. **320**(1): p. 64-71.

257. Akerman, S., H. Kaube, and P.J. Goadsby, *Anandamide is able to inhibit trigeminal neurons using an in vivo model of trigeminovascular-mediated nociception.* J Pharmacol Exp Ther, 2004. **309**(1): p. 56-63.

258. Akerman, S., H. Kaube, and P.J. Goadsby, *Anandamide acts as a vasodilator of dural blood vessels in vivo by activating TRPV1 receptors.* Br J Pharmacol, 2004. **142**(8): p. 1354-60.

259. Akerman, S., et al., *Endocannabinoids in the brainstem modulate dural trigeminovascular nociceptive traffic via CB1 and "triptan" receptors: implications in migraine.* J Neurosci, 2013. **33**(37): p. 14869-77.

260. Ashina, M., et al., *Migraine and the trigeminovascular system-40 years and counting.* Lancet Neurol, 2019. **18**(8): p. 795-804.

261. Russo, E.B., *Clinical Endocannabinoid Deficiency Reconsidered: Current Research Supports the Theory in Migraine, Fibromyalgia, Irritable Bowel, and Other Treatment-Resistant Syndromes.* Cannabis Cannabinoid Res, 2016. **1**(1): p. 154-165.

262. Sarchielli, P., et al., *Endocannabinoids in chronic migraine: CSF findings suggest a system failure.* Neuropsychopharmacology, 2007. **32**(6): p. 1384-90.

263. Osler, W.a.M.T., *Principles and Practices of Medicine.* 8 ed. 1916, New York: D. Appleton and Co.

264. Noyes, R., Jr. and D.A. Baram, *Cannabis analgesia.* Compr Psychiatry, 1974. **15**(6): p. 531-5.

265. Aviram, J., et al., *Migraine Frequency Decrease Following Prolonged Medical Cannabis Treatment: A Cross-Sectional Study.* Brain Sci, 2020. **10**(6).

266. Rhyne, D.N., et al., *Effects of Medical Marijuana on Migraine Headache Frequency in an Adult Population.* Pharmacotherapy, 2016. **36**(5): p. 505-10.

267. Stith, S.S., et al., *Alleviative effects of Cannabis flower on migraine and headache.* J Integr Med, 2020. **18**(5): p. 416-424.

268. Pini, L.A., et al., *Nabilone for the treatment of medication overuse headache: results of a preliminary double-blind, active-controlled, randomized trial.* J Headache Pain, 2012. **13**(8): p. 677-84.

269. Schindler, E.A.D., et al., *Exploratory investigation of a patient-informed low-dose psilocybin pulse regimen in the suppression of cluster headache: Results from a randomized, double-blind, placebo-controlled trial.* Headache, 2022. **62**(10): p. 1383-1394.

270. Abenhaim, H.A., et al., *Menopausal Hormone Therapy Formulation and Breast Cancer Risk.* Obstet Gynecol, 2022. **139**(6): p. 1103-1110.

271. Malfitano, A.M., et al., *Update on the endocannabinoid system as an anticancer target.* Expert Opin Ther Targets, 2011. **15**(3): p. 297-308.

272. Caffarel, M.M., et al., *Cannabinoids: a new hope for breast cancer therapy?* Cancer Treat Rev, 2012. **38**(7): p. 911-8.

273. Ellison, G.L., et al., *The National Cancer Institute and Cannabis and Cannabinoids Research.* J Natl Cancer Inst Monogr, 2021. **2021**(58): p. 35-38.

274. Fuhrman, B.J., et al., *Estrogen metabolism and risk of breast cancer in postmenopausal women.* J Natl Cancer Inst, 2012. **104**(4): p. 326-39.

275. Bab, I. and A. Zimmer, *Cannabinoid receptors and the regulation of bone mass.* Br J Pharmacol, 2008. **153**(2): p. 182-8.

276. Grodstein, F., et al., *Postmenopausal hormone therapy and risk of cardiovascular disease and hip fracture in a cohort of Swedish women.* Epidemiology, 1999. **10**(5): p. 476-80.

277. Kogan, N.M., et al., *Cannabidiol, a Major Non-Psychotropic Cannabis Constituent Enhances Fracture Healing and Stimulates Lysyl Hydroxylase Activity in Osteoblasts.* J Bone Miner Res, 2015. **30**(10): p. 1905-13.

278. Kang, M.A., J. Lee, and S.H. Park, *Cannabidiol induces osteoblast differentiation via angiopoietin1 and p38 MAPK.* Environ Toxicol, 2020. **35**(12): p. 1318-1325.

279. Desai, S., et al., *A Systematic Review and Meta-Analysis on the Effects of Exercise on the Endocannabinoid System.* Cannabis Cannabinoid Res, 2022. **7**(4): p. 388-408.

280. Gao, F., et al., *Signaling Mechanism of Cannabinoid Receptor-2 Activation-Induced beta-Endorphin Release.* Mol Neurobiol, 2016. **53**(6): p. 3616-3625.

281. Ibrahim, M.M., et al., *CB2 cannabinoid receptor activation produces antinociception by stimulating peripheral release of endogenous opioids.* Proc Natl Acad Sci U S A, 2005. **102**(8): p. 3093-8.

282. Cichewicz, D.L., *Synergistic interactions between cannabinoid and opioid analgesics.* Life Sci, 2004. **74**(11): p. 1317-24.

283. Cichewicz, D.L. and E.A. McCarthy, *Antinociceptive synergy between delta(9)-tetrahydrocannabinol and opioids after oral administration.* J Pharmacol Exp Ther, 2003. **304**(3): p. 1010-5.

284. Lee, M., et al., *A comprehensive review of opioid-induced hyperalgesia.* Pain Physician, 2011. **14**(2): p. 145-61.

285. Ibrahim, M.P., F; Lai, J. Albrecht, PJ; Rice, FL; Khodorova, A. et al., *CB2 Cannabinoid receptor activation produces antinociception by stimulating peripheral release of endogenous opioids.* Proceedings of the National Academy of Science, 2005. **102**: p. 3093-3098.

286. Guindon, J. and A.G. Hohmann, *The endocannabinoid system and pain.* CNS Neurol Disord Drug Targets, 2009. **8**(6): p. 403-21.

287. MacCallum, C.A. and E.B. Russo, *Practical considerations in medical cannabis administration and dosing.* Eur J Intern Med, 2018. **49**: p. 12-19.

288. Abrams, D.I., et al., *Cannabinoid-opioid interaction in chronic pain.* Clin Pharmacol Ther, 2011. **90**(6): p. 844-51.

289. Carter, G.T., et al., *Cannabis in palliative medicine: improving care and reducing opioid-related morbidity.* Am J Hosp Palliat Care, 2011. **28**(5): p. 297-303.

290. Seyfried, O. and J. Hester, *Opioids and endocrine dysfunction.* Br J Pain, 2012. **6**(1): p. 17-24.

291. Benyamin, R., et al., *Opioid complications and side effects.* Pain Physician, 2008. **11**(2 Suppl): p. S105-20.

292. Nguyen, T., et al., *Changes in Prescribed Opioid Dosages Among Patients Receiving Medical Cannabis for Chronic Pain, New York State, 2017-2019.* JAMA Netw Open, 2023. **6**(1): p. e2254573.

293. Patetsos, E. and E. Horjales-Araujo, *Treating Chronic Pain with SSRIs: What Do We Know?* Pain Res Manag, 2016. **2016**: p. 2020915.

294. Lape, E.C., et al., *Benzodiazepine Use and Dependence in Relation to Chronic Pain Intensity and Pain Catastrophizing.* J Pain, 2023. **24**(2): p. 345-355.

295. Gowers, W., *A Manual of Diseases of the Nervous System.* 1888, Philadelphia, PA: P. Blakiston Son and Co. .

296. Dauer, W. and S. Przedborski, *Parkinson's disease: mechanisms and models.* Neuron, 2003. **39**(6): p. 889-909.

297. Ajalin, R.M., et al., *Cannabinoid Receptor Type 1 in Parkinson's Disease: A Positron Emission Tomography Study with [(18) F]FMPEP-d(2).* Mov Disord, 2022. **37**(8): p. 1673-1682.

298. Venderova, K., et al., *Survey on cannabis use in Parkinson's disease: subjective improvement of motor symptoms.* Mov Disord, 2004. **19**(9): p. 1102-6.

299. Shohet, A., et al., *Effect of medical cannabis on thermal quantitative measurements of pain in patients with Parkinson's disease.* Eur J Pain, 2017. **21**(3): p. 486-493.

300. Lotan, I., et al., *Cannabis (medical marijuana) treatment for motor and non-motor symptoms of Parkinson disease: an open-label observational study.* Clin Neuropharmacol, 2014. **37**(2): p. 41-4.

301. Parkinson, J., *An essay on the shaking palsy. 1817.* J Neuropsychiatry Clin Neurosci, 2002. **14**(2): p. 223-36; discussion 222.

302. Postuma, R.B., et al., *Risk and predictors of dementia and parkinsonism in idiopathic REM sleep behaviour disorder: a multicentre study.* Brain, 2019. **142**(3): p. 744-759.

303. Prakash, S. and W.G. Carter, *The Neuroprotective Effects of Cannabis-Derived Phytocannabinoids and Resveratrol in Parkinson's Disease: A Systematic Literature Review of Pre-Clinical Studies.* Brain Sci, 2021. **11**(12).

304. Vuic, B., et al., *Cannabinoid CB2 Receptors in Neurodegenerative Proteinopathies: New Insights and Therapeutic Potential.* Biomedicines, 2022. **10**(12).

305. Kuo, H.C., et al., *Hericium erinaceus mycelium and its isolated erinacine A protection from MPTP-induced neurotoxicity through the ER stress, triggering an apoptosis cascade.* J Transl Med, 2016. **14**: p. 78.

306. Romigi, A., et al., *Cerebrospinal fluid levels of the endocannabinoid anandamide are reduced in patients with untreated newly diagnosed temporal lobe epilepsy.* Epilepsia, 2010. **51**(5): p. 768-72.

307. Mechoulam, R., *Interview with Prof. Raphael Mechoulam, codiscoverer of THC.. Interview by Stanley Einstein.* Int J Addict, 1986. **21**(4-5): p. 579-87.

308. McMeens, R., *Cannabis indica in convulsion.* Western Lancet, 1856: p. 327-331.

309. Lozano, I., *The therapeutic use of Cannabis sativa, L in Arabic Medicine.* Journal of Cannabis Therapeutics, 2001. **1**: p. 63-70.

310. Scheffer, I.E., et al., *Add-on cannabidiol in patients with Dravet syndrome: Results of a long-term open-label extension trial.* Epilepsia, 2021. **62**(10): p. 2505-2517.

311. Porter, B.E. and C. Jacobson, *Report of a parent survey of cannabidiol-enriched cannabis use in pediatric treatment-resistant epilepsy.* Epilepsy Behav, 2013. **29**(3): p. 574-7.

312. Sexton, M. *Towards a Medical Ethnography of Cannabis and Pediatric Epilepsy.* in *2018 Symposium on the Cannabinoids; International Cannabinoid Research Society.* 2014. Baveno, Italy.

313. Abrams, D.I. and M. Guzman, *Cannabis in cancer care.* Clin Pharmacol Ther, 2015. **97**(6): p. 575-86.

314. Parolaro, D., et al., *Endocannabinoids in the immune system and cancer.* Prostaglandins Leukot Essent Fatty Acids, 2002. **66**(2-3): p. 319-32.

315. Patsos, H.A., et al., *Cannabinoids and cancer: potential for colorectal cancer therapy.* Biochem Soc Trans, 2005. **33**(Pt 4): p. 712-4.

316. McAllister, S.D., et al., *Cannabinoids selectively inhibit proliferation and induce death of cultured human glioblastoma multiforme cells.* J Neurooncol, 2005. **74**(1): p. 31-40.

317. Guzman, M., et al., *A pilot clinical study of Delta9-tetrahydrocannabinol in patients with recurrent glioblastoma multiforme.* Br J Cancer, 2006. **95**(2): p. 197-203.

318. Twelves, C., et al., *A phase 1b randomised, placebo-controlled trial of nabiximols cannabinoid oromucosal spray with temozolomide in patients with recurrent glioblastoma.* Br J Cancer, 2021. **124**(8): p. 1379-1387.

319. Kabat-Zinn, J., *Full Catastrophe Living: Using the Wisdom of Your Body and Mind to Face Stress, Pain and Illness.* 1990, 2013, New York: Bantam.

320. Garrison, K.A., et al., *Meditation leads to reduced default mode network activity beyond an active task.* Cogn Affect Behav Neurosci, 2015. **15**(3): p. 712-20.

321. Miyazawa, M. and C. Yamafuji, *Inhibition of acetylcholinesterase activity by bicyclic monoterpenoids.* J Agric Food Chem, 2005. **53**(5): p. 1765-8.

322. Jiang, C.H., et al., *Anticancer Activity and Mechanism of Xanthohumol: A Prenylated Flavonoid From Hops (Humulus lupulus L.).* Front Pharmacol, 2018. **9**: p. 530.

323. Harish, V., et al., *Xanthohumol for Human Malignancies: Chemistry, Pharmacokinetics and Molecular Targets.* Int J Mol Sci, 2021. **22**(9).

324. Wang, K., et al., *Polysaccharopeptide from Trametes versicolor blocks inflammatory osteoarthritis pain-morphine tolerance effects via activating cannabinoid type 2 receptor.* Int J Biol Macromol, 2019. **126**: p. 805-810.

325. Habtemariam, S., *Trametes versicolor (Synn. Coriolus versicolor) Polysaccharides in Cancer Therapy: Targets and Efficacy.* Biomedicines, 2020. **8**(5).

326. Benson, K.F., et al., *The mycelium of the Trametes versicolor (Turkey tail) mushroom and its fermented substrate each show potent and complementary immune activating properties in vitro.* BMC Complement Altern Med, 2019. **19**(1): p. 342.

327. Sugawara, N., et al., *Lithium in tap water and suicide mortality in Japan.* Int J Environ Res Public Health, 2013. **10**(11): p. 6044-8.

328. Schrauzer, G.N., K.P. Shrestha, and M.F. Flores-Arce, *Lithium in scalp hair of adults, students, and violent criminals. Effects of supplementation and evidence for interactions of lithium with vitamin B12 and with other trace elements.* Biol Trace Elem Res, 1992. **34**(2): p. 161-76.

329. Pacholko, A.G. and L.K. Bekar, *Lithium orotate: A superior option for lithium therapy?* Brain Behav, 2021. **11**(8): p. e2262.

330. Wang, D., S.A. Jacobs, and J.Z. Tsien, *Targeting the NMDA receptor subunit NR2B for treating or preventing age-related memory decline.* Expert Opin Ther Targets, 2014. **18**(10): p. 1121-30.

331. Leo, M.S. and R.K. Sivamani, *Phytochemical modulation of the Akt/mTOR pathway and its potential use in cutaneous disease.* Arch Dermatol Res, 2014. **306**(10): p. 861-71.

332. Mandal, P.K., et al., *Cognitive Improvement with Glutathione Supplement in Alzheimer's Disease: A Way Forward.* J Alzheimers Dis, 2019. **68**(2): p. 531-535.

333. Mischley, L.K., et al., *Central nervous system uptake of intranasal glutathione in Parkinson's disease.* NPJ Parkinsons Dis, 2016. **2**: p. 16002.

334. Brakedal, B., et al., *The NADPARK study: A randomized phase I trial of nicotinamide riboside supplementation in Parkinson's disease.* Cell Metab, 2022. **34**(3): p. 396-407 e6.

Book Acronyms

2AG: 2-arachidonoylglycerol

AEA: arachidonoylethanolamide or anandamide

ACES: Adverse Childhood Experiences

AD: Alzheimer's Disease

APC: antigen presenting cell

BBB: blood brain barrier

BC : breast cancer

BDNF: brain derived neurotropic factor

BMD: bone mineral density

CB1R: Cannabinoid 1 receptor: found in the brain, on neurons, smooth muscle, endothelial cells

CB2R: Cannabinoid 2 receptor: found primarily in immune cells

CBD: cannabidiol

CBT: cognitive behavior therapy

CBR: cannabinoid receptor

CNR1/CNR2: these are the names of the genes that encode for CB1R and CB2R

COMT: catechol-O-methyltransferase: enzyme degrading dopamine, epinephrine, and norepinephrine

CSF: cerebrospinal fluid

CUD: cannabis use disorder

DA: dopamine

D2R: dopamine 2 receptor

DMN: Default Mode Network

EBV: Epstein barr virus

EC: endothelial cells- lining the inside of blood vessels

ECB: endocannabinoids: primarily AEA and 2AG

ECS: endocannabinoid system

EF: executive function

FAAH: fatty acid amide hydrolase: breaks down AEA

GABA: Gamma amino butyric acid, a neuroinhibitory neurotransmitter

GAD: generalized anxiety disorder

GPCR: G-protein coupled receptor

HIV: human immunodeficiency virus

HLA: human leukocyte antigen

HPA: Hypothalamic pituitary adrenal axix

HPG: Hypothalamic pituitary gut axis

HRT: hormone replacement therapy

HSA: hypothalamic spleen axis

MAG lipase: monoacylglycerol lipase- breaks down 2AG

MAO: monoamine oxidase: enzyme breaking down serotonin, melatonin, adrenaline, dopamine and more

MDMA: 3,4-Methylenedioxymethamphetamine

NAC: nucleus accumbens. Also, N-acetyl cysteine (an amino acid)

NGF: nerve growth factor

NK: Natural killer cells

NMDA: n-methyl-D-aspartate receptor

OC: oral contraceptive

PAMP: pathogen-associated molecular paterns

PCB: plant cannabinoid- cannabinoid compounds made by plants

PTSD: post-traumatic stress disorder

PD: Parkinson's Disease

RA: rheumatoid arthritis

ROS: reactive oxygen species

SNP: single nucleotide polymorphism

TBI: traumatic brain injury

THC: delta-9 tetrahydrocanabinol

TRPV1: transient receptor potential cation channel

VTA: ventral tegmental area

Acknowledgments

My primary motivation for writing this book lies in the intersection of studying botanical medicines and my love for providing women's healthcare. I have been a practitioner of both since 1994 when I became a certified herbalist, and then a Certified Professional Midwife. My Grandfather Dr. Ewell Hunt infused me with medical learning from childhood. When I told him that I was becoming a midwife, he passed his medical bag on to me before his death. He also used to attend home-births! Melanie Van Aken and Barbara Christman taught me midwifery and how to staunch a bad postpartum hemorrhage! Rosemary Gladstar was my first herbal teacher and Susan Sexton my first herbal and midwifery co-conspirator. An instructor in my horticulture education, Dr. Ellen Peffley, introduced me to the world of phytochemicals, piquing my interest in the biological activity of plant compounds. Dr. Nephi Stella at the University of Washington allowed me the opportunity to formally study the endocannabinoid system and get a good grasp on the pharmacology of cannabinoids. My Bastyr University instructors Dr. Eric Yarnell, Dr. Nancy Welliver and Dr. Robin DiPasquale deepened my love for, and understanding of, practicing botanical medicine.

I'm so grateful for all of the many women who have entrusted their stories to me. Thank you to the golden ones who trusted me for giving safe passage of their babies into the world and counseling them on natural health when no one else was available. For all of my patients who have been my teachers, may you be as enriched. My circle of women friends and family mean the world to me and I thank you all for your support as I ventured out of the comfortable world of my home and embarked on becoming who I fully am today. My utmost gratitude to LaJeune Wint, who achieved her mission by helping me reach my highest and best!

Thanks to Jahan Marcu, Nishi Whitely, Leah Belair, Mary Lynne Mathre, Genester Wilson-King, Mark Griffith, Donald Abrams, Terrie Best and Laurie Sexton McIntyre for looking over drafts plodding through proof-reads and taking precious time to give me feedback and guidance. And thanks to my brother Steve Sexton for hosting me in Taos and finally my partner Darryl Bornhop for relinquishing me for so many days of writing and his support in making this book a reality.

About the Author

D r. Sexton is an integrative medicine specialist and respected pioneer in the field of medical cannabis. She has over thirty years of experience as a midwife, herbalist, and naturopathic doctor. She is an expert in cannabinoid medicine and women's health across the lifespan. She formally studied the endocannabinoid system and its roles in health and illness, developed some of the first medical cannabis education for healthcare providers. She was an editor on the American Herbal Pharmacopoeia Cannabis Monograph and opened the first cannabis analytical lab in Washington State in 2010. She created Green Women's Guide, an online video learning experience, as a means to provide accurate information on cannabis and women's health for the general public.

Dr. Sexton practices medicine in California, speaks and teaches internationally and continues to develop her expertise on helping women heal.

www.ingramcontent.com/pod-product-compliance
Lightning Source LLC
Chambersburg PA
CBHW022047020426
42335CB00012B/583